For Gourmets with Ulcers

Toni Marsh Bruyère & Sidney Jean Robey

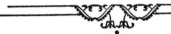

For Gourmets
with Ulcers

with Introductions by

Eric G. Schweiger, M.D. *and*

Robert L. Rowan, M.D., F.A.C.S.

W · W · NORTON & COMPANY · INC ·

NEW YORK

Contents

The Ulcer Patient
Eric G. Schweiger, M.D.   9

Understanding Ulcers
Robert L. Rowan, M.D., F.A.C.S.   13

Authors' Notes   15

Appetizers   21

Soups   31

Meats   41

Chicken and Other Poultry   67

Fish   91

Potatoes   103

Vegetables   115

Pasta and Rice   135

Eggs and Cheese   147

Salads   159

Desserts   173

Sauces   195

Shakes and Other Drinks   203

Canapés   211

Index   217

The Ulcer Patient

Recent surveys show that there are about 4,600,000 peptic ulcer patients in the United States. Duodenal ulcers are normally found to be four times as frequent as peptic ulcers. Those of us who treat peptic ulcers know there is no wonder drug to prevent or cure them, although many medications are useful in successful treatment.

Of course there are some fortunate individuals who, in spite of themselves, will recover from many ailments, but in general the ulcer is one disease that requires a high degree of cooperation from the patient. That is, he or she must accept and follow a doctor's advice in order to get well and stay well. To the patient it may seem as though the doctor is advocating a profound change in life-style, including eating habits, and very often this is actually so. But the patient who rebels, usually after prolonged and often favorable treatment, and then goes on a fried food-martini spree, is the one who can—*not* to his doctor's surprise—end up with a relapse.

One of the pressures the patient must learn to cope with while on an ulcer diet, is the urging of well-meaning friends and associates to go off the diet "just this one time." The ulcer patient should try to learn to decline with grace, to exercise self-discipline, and never to feel sorry for himself.

Another problem ulcer patients seem to worry about, often needlessly, is weight gain. It has been known to happen, of course, but very few people gain an unacceptable amount of poundage while on an ulcer diet. If the patient is concerned about figure control, he should take small but frequent portions, eat slowly, and realize that there is no need to finish absolutely everything on the plate. The ulcer dieter should try to remember that freedom from pain—whether nagging or intense—plus improved energy, strength, and eventual healing, are the rewards for sticking to a proper diet.

There are many ways a woman can be of significant help to her husband in the general and dietary aspects of ulcer therapy.

Maintain a relaxed and warm atmosphere in the home. The man without an ulcer has, in our time, more than enough stress and tension in his work and life in general. The executive with long hours, diverse responsibilities, and an ulcer, has an urgent problem that he can best learn to cope with in a calm, friendly home setting.

See to it that your husband has a short time to relax and regain his equilibrium when he comes home from work. Don't bring up complaints or ask for solutions at the dinner table.

Learn to prepare meals that are safe for the ulcerated stomach and provide a high level of satisfaction. Ulcer-diet blues (boredom with the diet) is a complaint so common that the doctor can virtually write it on the patient's chart before hearing it expressed.

A physical checkup, twice a year or as the doctor directs, is a necessity. A good doctor-patient relationship is of importance.

In *For Gourmets with Ulcers* Mrs. Bruyère and Mrs. Robey have taken the basic ulcer-food program of non-irritating and non-acid-producing foodstuffs, and assembled a collection of recipes that are nutritionally sound and intrinsically appealing. As this book provides a maintenance diet for the person with a healed peptic ulcer, it should be of considerable help and practical value to anyone who has an ulcer problem in the family.

Eric G. Schweiger, M.D.

Understanding Ulcers

There is no complete knowledge or understanding of the etiology of ulcers. There are certain factors that play an important part in the development of the ulcer, whether peptic or duodenal, but even these determining elements are not common to all ulcers. Increased acid secretion, digestive enzymes, emotional stress, as well as inborn resistance to these factors within the walls of the involved organs all play a varying role. No matter which of these causes is most prevalent, the significance of the patient's dietary intake is obvious. The organs that are diseased are the instruments of food digestion and what they are called upon to digest influences their function, health, and well-being.

Doctors vary in the method of treatment, depending upon the type of ulcer, its length of existence, the type of patient, and the patient's personality. Some physicians place great emphasis on the psychosomatic aspects of the disease; others do not stress this part of treatment. There is little difference of opinion, however, with regard to the following factors: Adequate rest, both physical and mental, is of value. Discontinuance of smoking and abstinence from acid-producing

13

alcoholic beverages are important. And diet directed toward the elimination of those foods that irritate and unwisely stimulate the digestive tract is a necessity. In fact, proper diet is an integral part of ulcer treatment.

Inasmuch as the main object of ulcer treatment is to heal the ulcer—and keep it healed—the reader will understand why cooking in a manner that encourages the patient to maintain the correct diet serves a purpose of inestimable value.

In this book, Mrs. Bruyère and Mrs. Robey have kept to this high purpose without forgetting that food should be more than merely safe, non-acid producing filler. It should be nutritious and entice both the eye and the appetite. These fine cooks prove that the required ulcer diet need not be tiresome to prepare nor boring for the patient—or the rest of the family—to eat.

If you face the dilemma of preparing food that is to be digested by an ulcer patient—and care about cooking—*For Gourmets with Ulcers* should be an essential handbook for problem-free eating, and a welcome addition to your cookbook collection.

Robert L. Rowan, M.D., F.A.C.S.

Authors' Notes

Is there an ulcer in your house? Is the patient bored to the point of rebellion with the ulcer diet? Are you, whether patient or cook, frustrated by the limitations of ulcer-diet menu planning—and weary of preparing separate meals for the other members of the family? If so, this book has been planned for you. The title may surprise you, but we hope the contents will prove that bland does not have to be blah, and that cooking for an ulcer patient does not mean an end to gourmet cooking.

Our book is a practical and realistic guide for the one who cooks for an ulcer graduate. By "ulcer graduate" we mean the patient who is well on the way to recovery, eating solid foods, and eager to return to a way of life that is as normal as possible.

The idea for the book came about when one of us had to meet the challenge of cooking for a food-conscious French husband who developed an ulcer. Happily we can report that ten years later the gentleman in question is not only in good health but slim as well. The other author, who attended Cordon Bleu classes in France, was an editorial associate, with experience in virtually all types of women's service copy at *Family Circle* magazine for ten years.

In selecting and developing our recipes, we have paid careful attention to the type of person most prone to peptic or duodenal ulcers. Actually, anyone—men and women of any age, teenagers, *outwardly* happy-go-lucky types, as well as high-strung individuals—can develop ulcers. However, the typical ulcer patient is an urban male between 35 and 50. The ulcer personality is usually described as sensitive, anxious, inner-directed, animated, moody, conscientious about work, and often holds a job that requires sociability. Obviously such a person is going to be thoroughly depressed by a seemingly endless regime of ground meat, puréed vegetables, and puddings. Who wouldn't be?

Ingenuity is the key word for the one who cooks for an ulcer graduate. She will probably find that her patient simply *cannot* digest some of the foods listed on the medical diet lists; and that he can indeed digest some of the foods mentioned as marginal or to be avoided. In view of this, we have included a few recipes for marginal foods, such as veal, in order to give our readers as much scope as possible. The ulcer patient may not be able to have spice, but he can and should have variety! You will find, however, that we have made a special notation on every recipe we think should be approached with some degree of caution.

To further complicate the life of the cook, a good many ulcer patients seem to develop an intense interest in food. They concern themselves not only with digestibility but with what others will think if they are given "different" foods. It is probably just human nature that, after a long period of strict ulcer dieting, even the person who has never before thought about his stomach suddenly becomes "involved" in what goes into his digestive system.

What actually does the doctor mean when he tells the ulcer patient that he must use discretion in his diet? Quite simply it means that the ulcer patient must not eat fried foods; sautéed meats and vegetables; highly seasoned sauces; browned butter and/or fat sauces; spices in virtually all forms; shellfish; pies, cakes, pastries; delicatessen sandwiches; and the roughage foods, such as salad greens, raw vegetables, raw fruits, and nuts. Does that sound like nearly everything in your culinary repertoire? If so, let's not get tense about the forbidden foods—and stay relaxed about all the foods an ulcer patient *can* eat.

This mission is not impossible, and our book proves the point, if the chef is willing to change some of her cooking techniques. In the following paragraphs we offer some concrete suggestions as to how the reader can alter her cooking methods and begin to prepare gourmet food that will please the most delicate stomach and the most discriminating palate.

Put away your frying pans. One of the most important rules in preparing food that is to go into an ulcerated stomach is to avoid fried foods.

A blender is an essential piece of kitchen equipment, not just a gadget, for the ulcer-diet cook. It need not be an expensive model with a complicated set of switches to fuss with, but a simple two-speed blender is a necessity for puréeing and breaking down some foods that otherwise might cause trouble.

You will find life as an ulcer-diet cook easier if you own several double boilers in various sizes. There are certain ulcer-diet cooking techniques—melting butter for example—that require the use of this type of pot, and having more than one will come in handy. Many of our recipes call for this piece of equipment.

Take down the spice rack, and put the condiments (pickles, catsup, mustard, Worcestershire sauce, and such) where they present no temptation to the patient. Do remember this: Fresh lemon juice can pep up many dishes, especially vegetables, and is a good substitute for pepper and other seasonings.

In some of our recipes you will find small amounts of wine or liquor. Although spirits evaporate rapidly in cooking, we do *not* recommend these recipes for those just going on to solid foods. However, a quarter of a cup of good wine added to a dish that will cook for some length of time can do a lot, psychotherapeutically, to help the post-ulcer patient feel less like a semi-invalid in an upright position. So, after careful consideration, we are including these recipes as our "lilacs for the soul."

Anyone who has ever been through a dangerous and lasting digestive upset must have engraved on his or her mind (or duodenum) that straight alcohol and/or cocktails can seriously upset a sensitive stomach. But, it is also a fact of life that, once free from painful symptoms, the ulcer type generally flatly refuses to give up social drinking entirely. For this reason—and because we want this book to be realistic and helpful to the reader—we have included a short chapter on canapés. These are cocktail snacks that can be served to guests, without advertising that the host (or hostess) has an ulcer.

When weight control or cholesterol control are elements to be considered, margarine can always be substituted for butter in our recipes. Fat-free milk can be used instead of whole milk, and low-fat cottage cheese in place of regular cottage cheese. In the few recipes calling for small amounts of pure olive oil, polyunsaturated oil can be used. All of our recipes have been tested with the substitute ingredients, as well as with butter, whole milk, and high quality olive oil.

In the introductory material to the various chapters you will find certain hints and information useful in preparing reaction-free and compliment-winning meals for the ulcer dieter. At the same time, we presume our readers have basic cooking skills. We believe that virtually all experienced cooks will know that a dish should be left uncovered, unless "cover" is specifically stated in the recipe.

For Gourmets with Ulcers does not perform the function of an elementary cookbook, nor is it a medical book. All of our recipes have been carefully tested, and none calls for foods or ingredients not listed as acceptable on standard ulcer-diet food lists. Nevertheless, when in doubt, the patient's doctor is always the best adviser.

After you have been using our book, we think you will find that you do not have to make separate meals for the rest of the family. Life being what it is, few women have the time or energy (and it's expensive too) to make different dishes for various members of the family.

Therefore, while we must tell you to put away the frying pans, the beloved spice rack, and the exotic casserole cookbook—at least for a while—we think we can help you get back to cooking one meal for the whole family—a meal that all will enjoy, including the one with the delicate stomach.

The authors are especially grateful to Dr. Eric G. Schweiger and Dr. Robert L. Rowan for their guidance and enthusiasm.

Eric G. Schweiger, M.D., has practiced gastroenterology for over fifteen years, during which time he has treated hundreds of peptic ulcer patients. He is also the author of a paper on the value of one of the therapeutic food supplements used in the early stages of peptic ulcer treatment.

Robert L. Rowan, M.D., F.A.C.S., is a urologic surgeon on the staffs of St. Vincent's Hospital of New York City and Columbus Hospital, New York City. Dr. Rowan was formerly a member of the research division of the Schering Corporation, where he worked on developing and monitoring new drugs. He has written approximately thirty scientific articles and is the author of *Horizontal Exercises*.

Our special thanks, too, go to Carol Houck Smith of W. W. Norton & Company, Inc., for her warm support and skillful editing.

And in conclusion, we must thank our respective husbands for their patience and encouragement, and for cheerfully taste-testing hundreds of recipes.

Sidney Jean Robey
Smoke Rise, New Jersey
December, 1970

Toni Marsh Bruyère
New York City
December, 1970

Appetizers

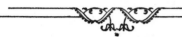

In these calorie-counting times, appetizers are generally not served at everyday family dinners. Nevertheless, when company comes, or on special occasions, an appetizer rather than soup is a festive beginning to a meal.

The usual appetizers—shrimp, crabmeat, mussels, stuffed clams, mushrooms, stuffed celery, spicy eggplant, rich patés, hors d'oeuvres variés—are not suitable for a troubled stomach. However, we have developed eleven recipes for appetizers that can be served to company with pride—and to the ulcer patient with confidence.

Keep the portions small. A good first course is meant to tantalize the appetite, not dull it.

Open Apple Rarebit

4 to 6 Servings

2 to 3 apples
6 slices white bread
Butter

6 slices mild American
   cheese
Brown sugar

Peel, core, and slice apples thinly.

Toast bread, and spread each piece with butter. Lay cheese slices on the buttered toast, and cover with apple slices. Sprinkle with brown sugar, and put under broiler until the cheese is melted. Serve at once.

Great for brunch too.

Artichokes à la Moscow

4 Servings

4 small artichokes
Dash of lemon juice
1 small jar unsalted caviar
   (black or red)

2 hard-cooked eggs, finely
   chopped

Cook artichokes according to instructions on page 117. Drain and chill. Remove the first two layers of leaves. Trim bottoms, so artichokes stand firmly. Spread open the remaining leaves; scoop out choke, and discard.

Put a little lemon juice in the hollow of each artichoke, and fill with caviar. Sprinkle with chopped hard-cooked egg. Serve very cold.

Avocado Mousse

4 Servings

3 or 4 avocados (2 cups of pulp)
1 tablespoon lemon juice
Salt
1 tablespoon unflavored gelatin

¼ cup cold water
¼ cup boiling water
¾ cup heavy cream
½ cup our mayonnaise (page 197)

Peel avocados, and remove pits. Mash the avocado flesh with a silver or stainless-steel fork, then force through a fine sieve. You should have 2 cups of pulp. Then add lemon juice and salt to taste.

Soften the gelatin in ¼ cup cold water, then dissolve in ¼ cup boiling water. While gelatin is dissolving, whip the cream. Fold mayonnaise into the whipped cream.

Fold whipped cream and mayonnaise mixture into the avocado pulp, then fold in the dissolved gelatin. Turn into a 1-quart mold that has been rinsed in cold water, and chill for 3 hours. Unmold before serving.

Avocado Varié

4 Servings

2 avocados
1½ cups cold cooked tongue,
    finely chopped
1 teaspoon olive oil

1 teaspoon lemon juice
Salt
4 teaspoons our mayonnaise,
    (page 197)

Halve the avocados, and remove pits. Taking care not to damage the shells, scoop out the avocado meat from each half and mash with a silver or stainless-steel fork. Add the chopped tongue, olive oil, lemon juice, and salt to taste.

When well mixed, refill shells with the avocado-tongue mixture. For a really rich taste, top each half with a teaspoonful of our mayonnaise.

Céleri-Rave Hors d'Oeuvre

4 Servings

Celery root prepared in this fashion is a typically French appetizer. This vegetable may not be immediately available in small towns, but it can be bought at any good greengrocer in large metropolitan areas. Buy only firm crisp roots, cut away any leaves and root fibers, then scrub roots vigorously with a kitchen brush.

1½ pounds celery root or
   knob celery
3 tablespoons lemon juice

⅓ cup olive oil
Salt

Peel celery root, and cut into julienne strips. Cook in boiling salted water for 20 minutes, drain and cool. When celery root is room temperature, add lemon juice, olive oil, and salt to taste. Mix lightly but well. Marinate for 2 hours in refrigerator before serving.

Chicken Custard

4 Servings

This is an old-fashioned but different first course.

4 eggs
1 cup strong chicken broth

1 cup cream
Pinch of salt

Break 4 eggs into a blender, and blend for 15 seconds, until light and well mixed.

Scald together 1 cup chicken broth and 1 cup cream. (Do not allow to boil.) Taste for salt. Remove broth-and-cream mixture from heat, and slowly add eggs. Stir well, and pour into 4 custard cups. Set 4 custard cups in a pan of hot water; bake in 350° oven for 40 minutes, or until a silver knife inserted in the center of a custard cup comes out clean. Serve warm.

Chicken-Avocado Appetizer

4 Servings

2 avocados
1 cup cold cooked chicken, finely chopped
4 to 6 canned asparagus spears, cut into small pieces

2 teaspoons olive oil
2 teaspoons lemon juice
Salt
4 teaspoons our mayonnaise (page 197)

Halve the avocados, and remove pits. Without damaging the shells, scoop out avocado meat from the halves and mash with a silver or stainless-steel fork. Mix with the chicken and asparagus; add olive oil, lemon juice, and salt to taste.

Refill the avocado shells with chicken and asparagus mixture. Top each avocado half with a teaspoonful of our mayonnaise. Serve well chilled.

Chicken-Citron Mousse

4 to 6 Servings

1 package lemon gelatin
2 cups cold cooked chicken, finely chopped
Salt

2 egg whites
Our mayonnaise (page 197) as garnish

Prepare gelatin according to directions on package. Cool until gelatin begins to thicken. Add chicken and a dash of salt.

Beat egg whites until very stiff, and fold into gelatin mixture.

Rinse a 1-quart mold in cold water. Turn mixture into mold, and chill several hours until firm.

Unmold onto a lettuce-bordered platter, remembering that lettuce is for appearance only—except for those in the family not on an ulcer diet. Garnish with our mayonnaise if desired.

Alpine Appetizer

2 to 3 Servings

⅔ cup milk
⅔ cup breadcrumbs
½ cup mild American
   cheese, grated

2 tablespoons butter
Dash of salt
2 eggs, separated

Scald milk in a double boiler. Add breadcrumbs, cheese, butter, and salt. Stir in *unbeaten* egg yolks. Beat egg whites until stiff, and fold into mixture. Pour into individual buttered baking dishes, leaving room for expansion. Place in a pan of hot water, and bake in 325° oven for 30 to 45 minutes, until firm. Serve immediately.

Gazpacho Aspic

8 Servings

1 can tomato soup
½ cup cream cheese
1 tablespoon butter
¼ teaspoon salt

1 tablespoon unflavored
  gelatin
¼ cup cold water
3 tablespoons lemon juice
½ cup heavy cream, whipped

Heat the soup (undiluted), cheese, butter, and salt in top of double boiler until the cream cheese has softened. Soften gelatin in ¼ cup of cold water, and dissolve in the hot mixture. Add lemon juice. Cool until mixture starts to thicken. Whip cream, and fold into mixture. Turn into a mold that has been rinsed in cold water, and chill until firm. Unmold, and serve.

This aspic can also be served as a salad.

First-Course Stuffed Tomatoes

4 Servings

4 large, firm, ripe tomatoes
4 to 6 chicken livers
2 cups cooked tongue,
  chopped
½ cup breadcrumbs
4 tablespoons butter, melted

3 tablespoons commercial
  sour cream
Salt
¼ cup grated Parmesan
  cheese

Cut the tops off the tomatoes, and scoop out the pulp. Discard pulp, or save for use in soups. Rub the inside of each tomato with salt.

Broil chicken livers; then dice finely.

Combine the diced livers, chopped tongue, breadcrumbs, butter, and sour cream. Season with salt to taste. Fill the tomatoes with mixture, sprinkle with cheese, and broil at least 6 inches from heat for 15 to 20 minutes.

Soups

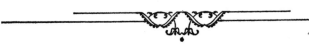

There are so many excellent canned, dehydrated, and frozen soups available in virtually every market that you should not have difficulty selecting those that will appeal to all family members and still be acceptable to the ulcer patient.

First, however, a word about Vichyssoise. Many people think this is a simple cold potato soup, and forget that it also contains leeks or onions—and therefore is not compatible with an ulcerated stomach.

Go easy also on the "hearty" soups. These are likely to contain too many forbidden ingredients for the ulcer graduate to handle with ease. Check all soup-can or box labels before buying.

Doctors and ulcer-diet food lists vary on the advisability of using consommé and beef or chicken broth as a soup base. Chemically speaking, soups produce acid, which the ulcer patient is trying to avoid. But cream or milk, when added to the soup, acts as an effective neutralizer. Therefore, in most of our recipes calling for a beef or chicken broth or consommé base, we also use cream or milk. A good rule to remember is that strong clear soups are for healthy stomachs.

As you probably know from your ulcer-diet sheet, oven-baked rolls, muffins, or biscuits should not be served. Toast made of a fine-textured white bread, melba toast, soda crackers, or water biscuits are agreeable substitutes with soup.

Avocado Soup

4 Servings

2 avocados
2½ cups clear chicken broth

1½ cups heavy cream
Dash of salt

Peel avocados, and remove pits. Mash the flesh of avocados with a silver or stainless-steel fork, then press the flesh through a fine sieve into a saucepan. Add chicken broth, and bring the soup to a boil. Reduce heat, and cook over a low flame, stirring occasionally, for 5 minutes. Stir in heavy cream, and taste for salt. Remove soup from fire, and chill thoroughly before serving.

Borscht in a Minute

6 Servings

1 can (16 ounces) beets
Liquid from beet can
2 cans beef bouillon

2 tablespoons lemon juice
Sour cream for topping

Drain beets, reserving the liquid from the can. Finely chop enough beets to make ¾ cup. Combine chopped beets, beet liquid, bouillon (undiluted), and lemon juice. Chill well.

Stir the borscht just before ladling into chilled cups or bowls. Top each serving with a dollop of sour cream.

Soup à la Grecque

---

6 Servings

2 cups clear chicken broth
1 cup cream
1 tablespoon cornstarch
3 egg yolks

Juice of 4 lemons
Salt
Lemon slices for garnish

Combine chicken broth and cream in a saucepan, and cook over low heat for 5 minutes, stirring constantly. Blend in cornstarch, and continue cooking over low heat until soup begins to thicken. Do *not* let mixture boil.

Beat egg yolks lightly, and gradually pour a little of the soup into them, stirring all the while. Then pour egg yolk mixture into the soup, and add lemon juice. Stir very well; add salt to taste.

Let soup cool, then chill overnight. Serve this soup very cold, garnished with a thin slice of lemon in each soup cup.

Consommé mit Ei

---

2 to 3 Servings

This is a very old European way of serving consommé.

1 egg per person

1 can beef consommé

Have eggs at room temperature. Dilute consommé, following directions on can. Heat soup to the boiling point, and pour into heated soup plates.

Break an egg into each plate, and cover immediately, so that the eggs get slightly poached. This must, of course, be done just before serving. At the table each person stirs the egg in his own bowl of soup.

Cucumber Soup

4 Servings

2 medium-size cucumbers
Dash of salt
2 tablespoons butter
2 tablespoons flour

2 cups clear chicken broth, approximately (you may need to add more)

Peel cucumbers, cut them lengthwise, and remove the seeds. Put the cucumbers into lightly salted boiling water, and simmer for 5 minutes. Drain, chop into small pieces, and set aside.

Melt butter in the top of a double boiler. Stir in the flour, and blend well. Add 2 cups chicken broth and the cooked, chopped cucumber. Stir very well, and cook in double boiler for 30 minutes.

Pour the soup into a blender, and blend for about 1 minute. Add salt if necessary. If soup seems too thick, add more broth now. Reheat the soup, and serve hot.

Summer Luncheon Soup

6 Servings

2 tablespoons unflavored
  gelatin
½ cup cold water
1½ cups boiling water
¾ cup cranberry juice

½ cup orange juice
¾ cup pineapple juice
2 tablespoons lemon juice
2½ tablespoons sugar
Salt

Soften the gelatin in cold water, then dissolve in boiling water. Add fruit juices, sugar, and salt to taste. Chill for several hours.

Before serving, break the jellied soup into small pieces by beating with a fork. Serve in tall thin glasses or bouillon cups.

Potato Soup à la Maison

2 Servings

Since commercial potato soups contain onions or leeks and spices, you may want to try this easy-to-prepare and easy-to-digest potato soup.

2¼ cups milk
2 large potatoes, boiled,
  peeled, and cubed
1 egg

½ tablespoon butter
¼ cup flour
Salt

Scald milk. Put scalded milk and all other ingredients into a blender, and blend for 1 minute. When completely smooth and blended, pour into saucepan, and heat over a low flame for 10 minutes, or until very hot.

St. Patrick's Soup

4 to 6 Servings

1 pound spinach
4 large potatoes, peeled
8 cups water

3 tablespoons olive oil
Salt

Wash and finely shred spinach. Set aside.

Cook potatoes in 8 cups boiling salted water until very tender, about 40 minutes. Remove potatoes, and keep the water in which they were cooked on low heat. Cut potatoes into small pieces, and place in a blender, along with about ½ cup of the cooking liquid. Blend 30 seconds or until smooth. Return puréed potatoes to pot of water.

Add shredded spinach, olive oil, and salt to taste to potatoes. Cook, uncovered, over high heat, stirring constantly for 3 minutes. Do *not* cook longer than 3 minutes, if you want soup to have a fresh green color.

Green Frappé (Cold Pea Soup)

6 Servings

Although many ulcer-diet food plans include green peas puréed in the third-stage diets, some ulcer patients can never tolerate peas. For those who *can,* this is one of the best pea soups ever.

1 package frozen green peas	1 cup heavy cream
1 cup water	Salt
1 cup clear chicken broth	

Cook peas according to directions on package, but use 1 cup water. When peas are very tender, pour in chicken broth.

Pour mixture into a blender, and mix for a few seconds until smooth. Add the heavy cream, and whirl the blender just a second or two. Taste for salt. Chill well before serving.

Cream of Spinach Soup

6 Servings

2 packages frozen chopped spinach, thawed and drained, but not cooked	2 teaspoons brown sugar
	3 cups clear chicken broth
	Salt
3 tablespoons butter	1 cup heavy cream

Put spinach, butter, brown sugar, and 1 cup of the chicken broth in a blender, and blend until the spinach is finely puréed and the mixture is smooth.

Pour into a saucepan, and add 2 more cups chicken broth. Cook over low heat for 10 minutes, stirring occasionally. Taste for salt.

Add cream, and heat thoroughly, but do not boil.

Cream of String Bean Soup

6 Servings

1 pound green string beans	½ cup sour cream
6 cups water	3 tablespoons lemon juice
3 egg yolks	Salt
3 tablespoons flour	

Use only tender, fresh, green string beans for this elegant and subtle soup. Wash beans, and remove loose strings. Cook in 6 cups boiling salted water until tender, about 30 minutes. Drain beans, but reserve all cooking liquid. Cut beans into ½-inch pieces, and set aside.

In a large mixing bowl, lightly beat egg yolks. Blend in flour, then add sour cream and lemon juice. Stir until mixture is smooth. Gradually add the reserved bean liquid and salt to taste. Stir very well to blend; pour mixture into a large saucepan.

Simmer soup over low heat, stirring constantly, until it thickens. Let soup cool, add cut-up beans, and chill at least 4 hours before serving.

Soup Alhambra

6 Servings

1 can cream of tomato soup
2 cups cream
2 teaspoons lemon juice

½ cup creamed cottage
   cheese
Salt

Combine the tomato soup (undiluted), cream, and lemon juice in a mixing bowl. Slowly beat with a rotary beater until well blended. Stir in cottage cheese and salt to taste. Chill. To serve, ladle into chilled bowls.

Tomato Polevka

4 Servings

1 tablespoon unflavored
   gelatin
½ cup cold water

2 cups tomato juice
Salt
Unsalted caviar for topping

Soften gelatin in cold water. Put 1 cup of the tomato juice in a saucepan; add softened gelatin, and heat until gelatin is dissolved. Add remaining tomato juice, and stir until well mixed. Add salt to taste.

Remove from heat, and pour into individual soup cups. Chill until fairly firm—about 2 hours. Top with a dollop of unsalted caviar before serving.

Meats

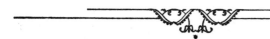

Meat is one of the most important elements in a meal, from the point of view of both nutrition and gratification. It contains protein for building and repairing body tissues, necessary iron, and riboflavin—a very important vitamin for those with digestive disturbances. This vitamin is also recommended to help depression and bring about a good mental outlook. It is obvious, therefore, that any cook will want to make the most out of her meat dishes.

The person who has had an ulcer soon becomes bored with plain boiled, broiled, and roasted meats, and has had these to distraction before the doctor allows him to venture into more sophisticated eating again. Our purpose is to put some adventure into ulcer-diet cooking, and you will find that there are plenty of interesting variations possible, even though the ulcer patient is not allowed pork and fried or sautéed meats.

All ulcer diet sheets allow beef and lamb, and some list veal as acceptable. The problem with veal is how to prepare it without resorting to the standard techniques of breading and frying, or sautéeing. Because veal is controversial, we are only listing three veal recipes—none of which calls for the use of a frying pan. Only the best veal is good enough for delicate stomachs, and the best quality is milk-fed veal. Unfortunately, much of the veal available in today's supermarkets is partial-grass or grain fed, and this meat can never have the tenderness of milk-fed veal. The best milk-fed veal is pale pink, not reddish in color.

Americans spend more money on meat than on any other food. It becomes therefore most important that the cook chooses first-quality non-sinewy meats. Of course, even good meats can be spoiled by improper cooking, so please be sure to follow our directions for cooking time and cooking heat.

Even if you have a favorite way of cooking roast beef, you might like to try this old-fashioned but sure-fire way to cook a roast. Put your meat in a 500° oven and cook it 5 minutes per pound for rare roast beef, 6 minutes per pound for medium. When that time is up, turn off the oven and leave the meat in the oven with the door closed for two hours. That's all. To avoid losing juices, and for easier carving, allow roasts (and meat loafs) to stand for 10 minutes after removing from the oven.

Steak Parmigiana

4 to 6 Servings

3 to 4 pounds sirloin or
   porterhouse
¼ cup olive oil
1 teaspoon lemon juice

½ cup grated Parmesan
   cheese
½ cup breadcrumbs
Salt

Put steak on a platter. Mix oil and lemon juice well, and pour over meat. Let marinate (not in the refrigerator) for 1 hour, turning a couple of times.

Blend cheese, breadcrumbs, and salt to taste.

Preheat broiler. Drain steak, *keeping marinade,* and put steak on broiler pan. Broil for 5 minutes. Remove from broiler, and quickly spread half the cheese mixture on the meat. Return to broiler, and broil until brown. Turn steak, and brush on a little of the marinade. Back to the broiler for 5 minutes, then quickly spread the rest of the cheese mixture on that side. Broil again until done.

This is a lot of in and out of the broiler, but the steak is quickly done and very savory.

Royal Bourbon Steak

6 Servings

This recipe takes over 2 hours to prepare.

Large sirloin steak (4 to 5 pounds), about 2 inches to 2½ inches thick

¼ cup bourbon (or more, depending on size of steak)

Trim off fat, and put the steak on a platter. Sprinkle 2 tablespoons of bourbon on each side, smoothing it over meat with the rounded side of a spoon, so that every bit of meat is covered. Leave standing for 1 hour.

Next, broil on both sides until brown—for this size steak, about 10 minutes on each side.

Remove from broiler, and place in a shallow roasting pan. Heat oven to 300°, and roast for 1 hour.

Remove steak to a warm platter. Slice and serve. The meat will be fairly well done, but delicious and tender.

Steak with Beef Marrow Sauce

6 Servings

¼ pound beef marrow (about 4 to 6 marrow bones)
Salt

4 tablespoons butter
½ cup dry white wine
3 pound sirloin steak

With the handle of a small spoon or fork push the marrow out of each bone. Put marrow in a small saucepan; cover with water, add a pinch of salt, and simmer for about 10 minutes. Drain well.

Melt the butter in the top of a double boiler. Add wine and a dash of salt. Cook over medium heat for 10 minutes. Add the marrow, mixing well. Keep warm.

Broil the steak as you usually do. When steak is ready, pour the hot sauce over it and serve.

Bohemian Beef

4 Servings

1 package soup greens (discard parsley and onion)	2 tablespoons water
	Salt
Grated rind of 1 lemon	½ pint plain yoghurt
2 pounds round steak	1 tablespoon lemon juice

Wash and carefully scrape the soup greens (carrots, celery, parsnip or turnip). Cut into small pieces. Grate rind of lemon, but do not mix into vegetables.

Broil—yes, broil—the round steak, just until pinkness disappears on both sides. Remove meat from broiler.

Put 2 tablespoons water, half of the cut-up vegetables, and salt to taste, in a Dutch oven or a heavy iron pot with a tight lid. Place the round steak on top of the vegetables, then put remaining vegetables over the steak. Sprinke on the grated lemon rind.

Cover, and bake in 375° oven for 30 minutes. After 30 minutes, give vegetables a stir to prevent sticking. Cover pot again, turn oven down to 350°, and continue cooking for another 30 minutes. Total cooking time, 1 hour.

Remove meat from oven, put on platter, and keep warm. Spoon out vegetables—you should have 2 cups of soft-cooked vegetables—and put in blender. Add ½ pint yoghurt and 1 tablespoon lemon juice. Blend for a few seconds until sauce is smooth. Slice meat into narrow strips, and pour sauce over all.

Steak Sandwiches

4 Sandwiches

¾ cup our Hollandaise
  Sauce (page 198)
4 small cube steaks, well
  cubed and pounded

4 slices white bread, toasted

Put Hollandaise in the top of a double boiler, and keep warm over very low heat. Do not let boiling water touch the top pan containing the sauce.

Broil the cube steaks, turning once. When steak is done as you like it, place each slice on a piece of toast, and spoon Hollandaise Sauce on top. Serve hot.

Boeuf en Gelée

6 Servings

3 to 3½ pounds beef
  eye-round roast
½ cup good burgundy wine
½ cup water

¼ cup cold water
½ teaspoon salt
1 teaspoon unflavored
  gelatin

Preheat oven to 325° for 10 minutes.

Set beef on a rack in roasting pan (do not add salt or water at this point), and roast in oven for 45 minutes.

Meanwhile, mix ½ cup good red wine with ½ cup water, and add salt. When meat has roasted for 45 minutes, pour wine mixture over the meat. Continue roasting (see time below), basting every 10 minutes with the wine mixture.

For 3-pound roast, cook: 20 minutes for rare; 35 minutes for medium.

For 3½-pound roast, cook: 30 minutes for rare; 40 minutes for medium.

When meat is done, remove from oven, and put in a shallow dish with sides. Skim off any fat from the beef-wine mixture in the roasting pan, then pour this mixture into a saucepan.

Soften gelatin in ¼ cup water, then add to beef-wine mixture. Cook over low heat, stirring constantly, until gelatin dissolves. Pour mixture over the meat. Let roast cool at room temperature, basting often with the wine-beef-gelatin mixture, until the meat has glazed. Chill in refrigerator.

Hawaiian Chuck Roast

6 to 8 Servings

3 to 4 pounds chuck roast
1½ cups grapefruit juice
1 tablespoon lemon juice
2½ cups pineapple juice

½ cup dry red wine
4 tablespoons butter, melted
Salt

Put chuck roast in a medium-size bowl. Mix all liquids and salt to taste; pour over roast. Marinate for 3 to 4 hours, turning now and then.

Take beef out of the marinade, keeping the liquid. Wipe meat dry, put in a roasting pan, and brown under broiler. Brush with butter to hasten browning.

Heat the marinade in a saucepan. Place beef in a Dutch oven or heavy casserole that has a lid, pour *half* the heated marinade over it, cover, and simmer for 2½ hours, adding more liquid as needed.

Remove cover, and roast another good half hour, until tender; then serve with rest of the marinade, which makes a delicious sauce.

Viennese Boiled Beef

6 Servings

This recipe is even better if made the day before serving.

3 carrots, sliced
6 stalks of celery, sliced
Salt

2 pounds chicken parts,
   (necks, back, and wings)
4 pounds brisket of beef

Combine sliced vegetables, salt to taste, and chicken parts in a pot. Add water to cover, bring to a boil, reduce heat, and simmer for 2 hours.

Put beef in a Dutch oven. Strain the vegetables and chicken stock over beef, discarding the chicken parts. Add more water, if needed, to cover meat. Cover the Dutch oven, and let beef simmer about 3 hours.

Our Basic Boeuf Bourguignon

6 Servings

2 packages soup greens
4 carrots
3 pounds chuck or stewing
   beef, cut into 1½-inch
   cubes
2 cans beef bouillon

2 cans tomato soup
Salt, if necessary
12 new potatoes
1 can (28 ounces) peeled
   tomatoes, drained

Wash and scrape all fresh vegetables except potatoes; cut into small pieces. Parsnips or turnip which come in soup-green packages must be sliced very thin. Discard parsley and onion.

Put beef, bouillon and tomato soups (undiluted), and all vegetables, except potatoes and tomatoes, in a large Dutch oven or a large heavy pot that has a tight lid. Bring to a boil, then reduce heat and simmer for 2 hours. Taste after cooking 30 minutes to see if salt should be added. (Bouillon usually eliminates the need for additional salt.)

Meanwhile, boil the potatoes. When done and cool enough to handle, peel.

After slowly cooking beef, vegetables, and soup mixture for 2 hours, add drained tomatoes and the cooked and peeled potatoes. Bring back to boil, reduce heat, and simmer for 5 to 10 minutes.

Drain off liquid, and serve as soup for first course. Serve beef and vegetables as main dish.

Minsk Beef

---

4 Servings

1½ pounds sirloin steak,
    cut into strips 2 inches
    long and ½ inch thick
2 tablespoons water

½ cup chicken broth
1 cup commercial sour
    cream
Salt

In a teflon pan or a heavy iron skillet put 2 tablespoons water and the meat. Cook over low heat for 5 to 10 minutes until the meat has lost its pinkness and is just slightly brown. Do not overcook.

Add chicken broth to meat. Cover, and cook for about 10 minutes over low heat. Uncover, and let liquid cook down for another 10 minutes. Add sour cream, mix well, and taste for salt. Keep on low fire until sour cream has heated. Do not boil. Serve on rice or noodles.

This is, of course, a variation of Beef Stroganoff, and very easy to make—but it requires a tender cut of beef.

Shepherd's Pie

---

3 to 4 Servings

2 cups cooked beef or lamb, cubed

1 cup mixed leftover vegetables, drained (string beans and carrots, for example)

2 cups cooked dehydrated mashed potatoes

¼ cup cream

1 egg, beaten

1 tablespoon butter

Preheat oven to 400°. Lightly butter a 1½-quart casserole. Place meat in casserole, and add drained vegetables.

Make 2 cups dehydrated mashed potato, following directions on box. Add cream.

Beat egg until light. Fold into the potato mixture. Spread mixture over meat and vegetables. Dot the top with butter. Bake 20 minutes, or until lightly brown.

Poorer-than-a-Shepherd Pie

---

3 to 4 Servings

1 tablespoon water

1¼ pounds lean ground round

Salt

2 cups cooked dehydrated mashed potatoes

2 tablespoons grated Parmesan cheese

1 tablespoon butter

Put 1 tablespoon water in a heavy skillet, add ground meat, and salt to taste. Cook over low heat until meat has lost its pinkness, but do not brown.

Make 2 cups dehydrated mashed potatoes following directions on box.

Place cooked ground meat in a lightly buttered casserole. Top with mashed potatoes, making a crust. Sprinkle with grated Parmesan cheese, and dot with butter. Bake in 375° oven for 30 minutes, until nicely browned.

Scandinavian Meat Ring

4 Servings

1½ pounds lean ground round	Salt to taste
¾ cup breadcrumbs	¾ cup club soda (never mind the questions, just try it)
3 eggs	

Mix all ingredients well, adding the soda last, until you get a nice mushy paste that hangs on the spoon but is still fairly pink (not gray).

Butter a 9-inch ring mold, spoon in mixture, and bake in 350° oven for about 45 minutes. To see if done, insert a skewer; it should come out clean.

Use a sharp knife to loosen before unmolding. This dish makes a lovely fluffy meat ring.

Meatballs Jutlandia

4 Servings

1½ pounds lean ground
    round
¾ cup breadcrumbs

3 eggs
Salt to taste
¾ cup club soda

As in the previous recipe, mix all ingredients well, adding the soda last, until you get a paste that hangs on the spoon but is still pinkish, not gray.

Once you have combined the ingredients to make a paste, put a large pot of salted water to boil. When the water is boiling, form small meatballs between your palms, and drop them one at a time into the water, being sure that the water comes back to boiling each time. Generally, the meatballs are done when they start rising to the surface of the water. To be sure, scoop one out, cut in half and see whether it is cooked through.

These meatballs can be served with Sauce Verte, page 198, or with tomato soup diluted with a little milk, and heated.

Made very small, Meatballs Jutlandia can also be served as an appetizer. Try broiling them for a minute on each side before serving on toothpicks.

Glazed Meat Loaf

6 Servings

1 pound lean ground round
1 egg
¼ cup milk
3 tablespoons tomato juice

Salt
3 orange slices
⅓ cup apple jelly
2 teaspoons hot water

Mix the ground beef, egg, milk, tomato juice, and salt to taste together in a mixing bowl. Lightly butter an 8½ x 4½ x 2½-inch loaf pan, and pack beef mixture in tightly. Run a knife around the sides of the pan, freeing the loaf from the sides just slightly. Bake in 400° oven for 1 hour. Remove from oven—but do not turn oven off. Let loaf stand for 5 minutes, then turn onto *oven-proof* platter. Arrange 3 orange slices over top.

Meanwhile, about 10 minutes before meat loaf is done, cook apple jelly and water over low heat until smooth. Spoon some of this glaze over loaf, and return to oven for 5 minutes. Then spoon more glaze on loaf. Leave in oven an additional 5 minutes.

Toni's Meat Loaf

4 to 6 Servings

1½ pounds lean ground round

3 eggs

1 can tomato soup, undiluted

1½ cups packaged herb-seasoned stuffing

Salt to taste

Mix ingredients well, and pack into a buttered loaf pan. Bake in 375° oven for ½ hour, then turn oven down to 350° and bake for another ½ hour. Total baking time: 1 hour. We recommend always making two meat loaves, and freezing one for later use.

The meat loaf can be served with additional tomato soup diluted with a little milk as sauce.

This recipe is not for those just going onto a normal diet, but the herb seasoning in the stuffing will not bother the average ulcer graduate.

Tipsy Hamburgers

4 Servings

1½ pounds lean ground round

3 tablespoons cognac

Preheat broiler. Form the meat into 4 patties, and place on broiling rack.

Brown on one side, remove from broiler, and turn the meat. Drizzle cognac on each patty, and return to broiler until meat is done to your taste.

The Most Agreeable Ground Beef

4 Servings

This recipe is simple to the point of being ridiculous, but grown men and little children love it.

2 tablespoons water
2 pounds lean ground round
4 tablespoons butter

4 tablespoons flour
2 cups milk
Salt

Put 2 tablespoons water in a heavy skillet. Add ground beef, and cook until pinkness disappears. Do not brown.

Melt butter in the top of a double boiler. When melted,

stir in flour and blend well. Add milk, and stir until the sauce is smooth and begins to thicken.

Add ground beef and salt to taste. Stir well, and let sit in double boiler over low heat for about 15 minutes. Stir before serving. (This dish will keep very well in the double boiler over low heat, should dinner be delayed.) Serve on rice or toast.

Beef-Noodle Casserole

6 Servings

1 box (8 ounces) noodles
1 tablespoon water
2½ pounds lean ground round
Salt

2 cans cream of mushroom soup
2 cups milk
Breadcrumbs
1 tablespoon butter

Cook noodles according to directions on box. Drain, and set aside.

Put 1 tablespoon water in a heavy iron skillet. Add ground meat and salt to taste. Cook over low fire until meat is lightly browned.

Put the soup and milk in a large bowl, and mix well. Fold in the noodles and the beef. Lightly butter a casserole, and transfer the mixture to it. Sprinkle with breadcrumbs, dot with butter, and bake in 350° oven for 30 minutes, or until lightly browned.

Beef Flamingo

4 Servings

4 large tomatoes
1 tablespoon water
1 pound lean ground round
Salt

1 cup cooked rice
4 teaspoons breadcrumbs
4 teaspoons butter

Wash, core, and scoop out tomatoes. Turn upside down to drain. (Keep left-over tomato pulp for use in soups.)

Put 1 tablespoon water in a heavy iron skillet; add meat, and cook until meat has lost its pinkness. Add salt to taste. Mix in 1 cup cooked rice, and combine thoroughly. Stuff tomatoes with this mixture. Top each tomato with 1 teaspoon breadcrumbs and 1 teaspoon butter. Bake in 375° oven for 35 minutes.

The ulcer patient must not eat the tomato skin.

Polynesian Medley

10 Servings

1 pound lean ground round
1 egg
¼ cup breadcrumbs
2 tablespoons milk
1 teaspoon salt
½ pound chicken livers, halved and cleaned of fat

1 can (14 ounces) pineapple chunks, with juice
¼ cup light brown sugar, firmly packed
2 tablespoons cornstarch
1 envelope instant chicken broth
3 tablespoons lemon juice

Combine ground beef, egg, breadcrumbs, milk, and salt in a medium-size bowl. Mix lightly until well blended. Shape into small balls.

Broil the meatballs, turning once, until well browned, and put in a large baking dish.

Broil chicken livers until they lose their pink color. When done, add to baking dish.

Drain syrup from the pineapple chunks into a 1-cup measure, add water if needed to make ¾ cup of liquid, and set aside. Add pineapple chunks to the baking dish.

Mix brown sugar, cornstarch, and powdered chicken broth in a small saucepan. Stir in the pineapple juice and 3 tablespoons lemon juice. Cook, stirring constantly, until sauce thickens and boils for 3 minutes. Pour over meats, and pineapple, and cover. Bake in 325° oven for 30 minutes to blend the flavors.

If you are serving this recipe at a party, keep it warm in a chafing dish.

Honey Gigot

4 to 6 Servings

¾ cup honey	3 tablespoons lemon juice
¼ cup light brown sugar	¼ teaspoon salt
1 tablespoon orange juice	Leg of lamb (5 to 6 pounds)

Combine the ingredients, except the lamb, and stir over low heat until blended. Put aside.

Cut as much fat off the lamb as possible, and roast in the oven in your usual way for approximately 2½ hours. We start at 375°, cutting down to 350° after about 45 minutes.

Half an hour before lamb is done, remove from oven and cut off the skin and fat. Drain fat from pan. Pour honey sauce over lamb, and return to oven for about 30 minutes, basting during that time.

Lamb en Brochette

2 Servings

2 lamb steaks per person
1 cup olive oil
Juice of ½ large lemon
Salt

10 to 12 small cherry
    tomatoes
1 can (8¼ ounces)
    pineapple wedges
4 metal skewers

Cut lamb into 1-inch squares, removing as much fat as possible. Combine oil, lemon juice, and salt to taste; pour over lamb chunks and let marinate at least 1 hour.

Drain lamb and arrange on skewers, alternating with tomatoes and chunks of drained pineapple. There should be enough of all ingredients for 4 medium-size skewers.

Place skewers on a broiling rack, and broil about 4 to 6 inches from heat for 10 to 15 minutes, turning at least once. Makes delicious kebabs, but the ulcer patient must remember not to eat the tomato skins.

Casserole d'Agneau

2 to 3 Servings

6 loin lamb chops
1 can (8½ ounces) small
    potatoes, drained
1 can (16 ounces) small
    Belgian carrots, drained

3 ripe peeled tomatoes,
    quartered
¾ cup consommé
Salt

Cut all the excess fat off lamb chops. Brown under broiler for a few minutes on each side.

Preheat oven to 350°.

Place the chops flat (not overlapping) in a buttered casserole that has a lid. Top with drained potatoes, carrots, and tomatoes. Add consommé.

Cover casserole, and bake for about 1 hour, or until the chops are tender. Add salt to taste.

Cranberry Ragout of Lamb

6 Servings

2 pounds lean boneless shoulder of lamb
2 teaspoons salt
½ cup cranberry-apple juice
½ cup cold water

1 package frozen green beans
2 medium-size yellow squashes, scraped and sliced
¼ cup flour
½ cup warm water

Trim fat from lamb, and cut into 1-inch cubes. Put in a Dutch oven; add salt, cranberry-apple juice, and ½ cup cold water. Cover, and bring to a boil. Reduce heat and simmer for 1 hour, or until meat is nearly tender.

Add vegetables, cover again, and simmer for 30 minutes, or until lamb and vegetables are tender.

Remove lamb and vegetables (retaining liquid), and put on a heated serving plate. Keep warm. Pour liquid into a 2-cup measure. If not enough, add water to make 2 cups, and return to Dutch oven.

Shake flour in an empty jar with ½ cup warm water until well blended, and add to liquid in Dutch oven. Cook, stirring constantly, until gravy thickens. Don't let it boil more than a minute. Now pour gravy over meat and vegetables, and serve.

Lamb and Macaroni Casserole

4 Servings

1 cup macaroni, cooked and drained
1 cup cooked lamb, finely chopped

Salt to taste
Few drops lemon juice
2 eggs, slightly beaten
1½ cups milk

Put the macaroni into a buttered casserole. Mix lamb, salt, and lemon juice; spread over the macaroni. Then mix the eggs and milk, and pour over ingredients in the casserole. Bake in 350° oven for 30 to 45 minutes, until firm. Insert a silver knife; if it comes out clean, the dish is done.

Lamb and Potatoes au Gratin

4 Servings

1½ cups cooked lamb, cubed
3 cups cooked potatoes, diced
4 tablespoons butter
3 tablespoons flour

2 cups milk
Salt
4 tablespoons grated mild American cheese
4 tablespoons breadcrumbs

Put lamb and potatoes in a 1½-quart baking dish.

Melt 3 tablespoons of the butter in the top of a double boiler. When melted, blend in flour. Gradually add milk, and continue cooking until sauce is smooth and thickened. Add salt to taste.

Pour sauce over lamb and potatoes. Sprinkle with grated cheese and breadcrumbs. Dot with remaining tablespoon butter. Bake in 400° oven for 30 minutes.

Lamb and Spinach Casserole

4 Servings

2 cups cooked lamb, cubed
2 packages frozen chopped
   spinach
4 tablespoons butter
4 tablespoons grated mild
   American cheese

Dash of sherry
4 tablespoons our
   mayonnaise (page 197)
Salt

Cut cooked meat into 1-inch cubes. Cook spinach according to directions on package. Drain. Combine all ingredients in a large bowl, and mix well. Spoon into a casserole, cover, and heat in 350° oven for about 30 minutes.

Lamb and Fruit Mold

6 Servings

1 can (11 ounces) mandarin
  orange segments
1 can (8¾ ounces)
  pineapple spears
Juice from both fruit cans
2 tablespoons unflavored
  gelatin
1 cup cold water
1½ cups boiling water

¾ cup sugar
½ cup lemon juice
Salt
1 cup cold cooked lean
  lamb, cut into small
  pieces
Our mayonnaise (page 197)
  for garnish

Drain orange segments and pineapple spears, and reserve juice from both cans.

Soak the gelatin in cold water for 5 minutes, then dissolve in boiling water. Remove from heat; add sugar, lemon juice, a dash of salt, and fruit juices from the cans. Stir very well, and chill.

When the mixture begins to thicken, fold in fruit and cut-up lamb. Turn into a 2-quart ring mold that has been rinsed in cold water. Chill until firm, about 3 to 4 hours. Unmold onto lettuce-bordered platter, remembering, of course, that lettuce is not for the ulcer dieter. Garnish with our mayonnaise, if desired.

Chicken-Stuffed Veal Roast

8 Servings

Check with your doctor and/or your ulcer-diet food list to see if veal is allowed. If so, this is an excellent way to roast it, especially for company meals.

Salt
1 veal shoulder (about 4 pounds) with pocket for stuffing
2 cups cooked chicken, finely minced
4 lightly broiled chicken livers, finely minced

1 cup grated Parmesan cheese
1/4 cup heavy cream
1 tablespoon olive oil
3/4 cup clear chicken broth
1/4 cup dry white wine

Rub salt over the veal, including inside the pocket. Mix together minced chicken and chicken livers, Parmesan cheese, and heavy cream. Spoon this mixture into the veal pocket. Close the pocket with small skewers, then tie the roast into a roll with string. Rub the surface of the veal with about 1 tablespoon olive oil.

Place in a roasting pan, and roast in 300° oven for 3½ hours. Baste occasionally with chicken broth. During the last 30 minutes, baste with dry white wine.

When meat is done, let stand 10 minutes before removing string and carving.

Hungarian Loaf

4 Servings

Please check your diet-food plan before cooking veal for an ulcer patient.

1½ pounds ground veal	1 cup breadcrumbs
2 cups grated raw carrots	Salt
1 cup commercial sour cream	

Mix all ingredients in a large mixing bowl. When well combined, turn into a lightly buttered loaf pan. Run a knife around the edges of the loaf to free it slightly from the sides of the pan. Bake in 350° oven for 1 hour, or until lightly browned on top.

Veal-Tuna Loaf with Chicken Noodle Sauce

4 Servings

Please check your diet-food plan before cooking veal for an ulcer patient.

2 cans (7 ounces each) tuna in water pack	½ cup breadcrumbs
1 pound ground veal	¾ cup milk
2 eggs	Salt
	1 can chicken noodle soup

Drain tuna, and combine with ground veal, eggs, bread-crumbs, and milk. Add salt to taste, and mix well.

Pack the mixture into a lightly buttered 4 x 8-inch loaf pan, and bake in a 350° oven for 1 hour and 30 minutes.

Serve the veal-tuna loaf with this good and easy-to-make sauce: Put chicken noodle soup (undiluted) in a blender. Blend until soup is smooth and has a sauce-like consistency. Pour into saucepan and heat over low flame until hot.

Lamb Kidneys Aloha

4 Servings

1 cup olive oil
Juice of 1 lemon
Salt

8 lamb kidneys
2 cans (8¼ ounces) sliced
    pineapple

Make a marinade of the oil, lemon juice, and salt to taste, and put in a large flat bowl.

Wash, dry, and split the kidneys down the middle length-wise. Remove fatty centers with a shape knife. Place kidney halves in the marinade, and let stand for at least 1 hour.

Drain pineapple slices. Discard marinade, and place 2 to 3 kidney halves on each slice of pineapple on broiler rack.

Broil about 4 inches from heat for 5 to 6 minutes; then remove from oven, and turn only the kidney halves. Return to broiler for another 5 to 6 minutes, until kidneys are done through.

Broiled Calf's Liver au Citron

4 Servings

2 tablespoons olive oil   1 teaspoon salt
3 teaspoons lemon juice   4 slices calf's liver

Mix the olive oil, lemon juice, and salt.

Wash the liver under running cold water, and dry on paper towel.

Place liver on broiler rack, and brush upper side with half the lemon-oil mixture. Broil liver until one side is done, then turn and brush the other side with remaining lemon-oil mixture. Return to broiler.

Serve with an additional squeeze of lemon juice on top, if desired. Lemon gives an added fillip to the liver taste.

Boiled Tomato Tongue

4 to 8 Servings, depending on size of tongue

1 package precooked tongue   ¾ cup milk
1 can tomato soup

Packaged precooked tongue is widely available, and is a good food for ulcer-diet patients. Follow the package directions for heating.

When the tongue is done, pierce the cellophane wrapper with a sharp knife, but slowly and carefully, otherwise the hot juice may squirt from the package. Drain the juice and discard.

Heat a can of tomato soup diluted with ¾ cup milk until hot. Slice the tongue for serving and use tomato soup as gravy.

Chicken and Other Poultry

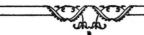

Chicken is usually a fairly economical buy and, aside from costing less than beef or lamb, it is an excellent source of protein and a very good source of vitamin B and calcium. Chicken also lends itself to all sorts of cooking variations, as you will see from the thirty recipes that follow.

Buy only tender, young chickens for ulcer-diet cooking. If you are serving a number of people and need more meat for your recipe, buy a capon. Cook chicken at low temperature (high-temperature cooking tends to dry out poultry), and serve it well done. Generally, we prefer to remove the skin before cooking. The skin is difficult to digest, and removing it cuts down on the fat content.

Very lean duck can be digested by those who have well-healed ulcers, but keep the portions small and the rest of the meal plain and simple.

Try serving applesauce with a dash of rum with broiled chicken. Raspberry sherbet also makes a festive side dish with roasted or broiled chicken. Serve plain rice with elaborate poultry recipes.

Fresh poultry should, of course, be cooked within two days after purchase.

Rumanian Roast Chicken

4 Servings

1 small roasting chicken
  (about 2 pounds)
Salt to taste

1 cup plain yoghurt
1 cup heavy cream

Wash and dry chicken, rub well with salt. Roast in 350° oven for 10 minutes.

Combine the yoghurt and heavy cream, and pour over chicken after 10 minutes' cooking time. Continue roasting, basting frequently with the sauce, for 1½ hours, or until chicken is tender.

The chicken skin should, of course, be removed from the portion served the ulcer patient.

Chicken with Peaches

4 to 6 Servings

2 small broilers, cut in
  serving pieces
Salt

5 tablespoons butter
1 can (14 ounces) peach
  halves, *with* juice

Put chicken in a single layer in a shallow baking pan. Sprinkle lightly with salt.

Melt butter in the top of a small double boiler. When melted, add ½ cup juice from the canned peaches. Heat for

5 minutes, then pour over chicken. Bake in 400° oven for 1 hour, basting occasionally.

During last 10 minutes, put drained peach halves around the chicken.

Sweet and Low Broiled Chicken

2 to 3 Servings

1 small broiler, cut in serving pieces	2 teaspoons salt
1 lemon	1 teaspoon sugar
¼ cup butter, melted	

Remove skin, and wash the chicken, wiping dry with paper towels. Rub each side with a cut lemon, squeezing to keep juice flowing. Roll chicken pieces in melted butter until all are well coated; sprinkle with salt. Then the crowning touch —a light sprinkling of granulated sugar.

Line a broiling pan with foil—or use a disposable pan—and coat with a little of the melted butter. Put the chicken pieces in the pan, round side down. Place about 4 inches from broiler heat, and brown for 10 minutes, turning once.

Lower pan to second-rack tier of broiler, and continue broiling for about 30 minutes, turning several times and basting with the pan juices.

If the sugar starts to burn, add a little water.

Pilau of Chicken

3 to 4 Servings

1 small broiler, cut in pieces
1 cup olive oil
Juice of 1 lemon
1 can tomato soup
1 can (16 ounces) whole
   peeled tomatoes
2 teaspoons butter

½ teaspoon salt
1 cup packaged precooked
   rice
¼ cup grated Parmesan
   cheese

Remove skin from chicken pieces. Make a marinade of the olive oil and lemon juice, and let chicken pieces marinate in mixture for 1 hour.

Preheat broiler. Drain chicken, discarding marinade, and wipe pieces with paper towel. Place chicken pieces on rack of broiler pan, and broil for 5 to 10 minutes on each side, until browned. Remove from broiler.

Pour tomato soup (undiluted) and can of whole peeled tomatoes into a large saucepan. With a sharp knife cut tomatoes in half. Add chicken pieces, and bring to a boil. Cover, and simmer for 30 to 40 minutes, until chicken is very tender. Turn off heat.

Pour off 1¾ cups of the tomato-chicken gravy, and put in separate saucepan. Add 2 teaspoons butter and ½ teaspoon salt, and bring to a boil. When boiling, take off heat, and add 1 cup packaged precooked rice. Cover, and let stand for 10 minutes, stirring once or twice.

Now add the rice to the chicken and rest of tomato gravy, and keep warm. When serving, sprinkle Parmesan cheese on top.

Chicken Stew Bruyère

8 Servings

2 chickens, broilers or fryers, cut in serving pieces
2 packages soup greens
4 carrots
2 cans beef bouillon
2 cans tomato soup

2 cups tomatoes, peeled and cut up
10 to 12 small new potatoes, boiled and peeled
Salt

Wash chicken pieces and remove skin.

Wash and scrape all vegetables, cut into small pieces or slices. Parsnip or turnip, which come in soup-green package, must be sliced very fine. Discard parsley and onion.

Put chicken pieces, all the soup (undiluted), the soup greens, and the carrots into a large Dutch oven or large heavy skillet with a lid. Bring to a boil, reduce heat, and simmer for about 1 hour. Add peeled and cut-up tomatoes and cooked, peeled potatoes. Bring back to boil and simmer, covered, for another 15 minutes. Add salt to taste.

Drain off liquid, and serve this as soup for a first course. Serve chicken and vegetables as your main dish.

Casserole Poulet aux Légumes

6 Servings

2 small broilers, cut in pieces and skinned
Salt
4 tablespoons butter, melted
About 1 cup boiling water

½ pound whole green beans, washed and cleaned
5 small carrots, scraped
8 to 10 very small new potatoes, peeled
½ cup clear chicken broth

Put chicken pieces in a large casserole that has a lid, sprinkle with salt to taste, and add melted butter. Pour in boiling water (it should be about 1-inch deep). Cover, and bake in 375° oven for 30 minutes.

Meanwhile, prepare vegetables as instructed above. Parboil for 10 minutes, and set aside.

After chicken has baked for 30 minutes, add parboiled vegetables and chicken broth. Continue baking for another 30 minutes, or until chicken is tender.

Chicken Capri

4 Servings

2½ pounds chicken, cut in
  pieces and skinned
3½ cups cut-up tomatoes,
  peeled

Salt
½ cup dry white wine
1 tablespoon flour

Broil chicken pieces for about 15 minutes, until browned lightly.

Cut up peeled tomatoes, add salt to taste, and put in a large heavy pot. Add chicken pieces, cover, and simmer for 45 minutes, until chicken is tender, and tomatoes thoroughly cooked. Add dry white wine during last 15 minutes.

If you wish to thicken the sauce slightly, you can add 1 tablespoon all-purpose flour, or use our European sauce-thickening method, page 197.

Beaumont Chicken Bake

4 Servings

3 chicken breasts
3½ cups lightly salted water
2 cups packaged, precooked
   rice
1 can chicken gravy

Salt
1 cup ready-mix bread
   stuffing
1 tablespoon butter

Boil chicken breasts (leaving skins on) in 3 cups lightly salted water, in a pot with a tight lid, for 25 minutes. Remove chicken from liquid, and let cool. Pour off 2 cups of broth to use when cooking the rice. When chicken is cool enough to handle, remove skin and take out bones. Cut the meat into small pieces.

Cook rice in 2 cups of chicken broth, following directions on box, adding water if necessary.

Heat chicken gravy in a small saucepan; add remaining ½ cup water. Add salt to taste.

Spoon rice into a baking dish, top with cut-up chicken, pour gravy over all. Sprinkle bread stuffing on top, and dot with 1 tablespoon butter. Bake in 400° oven for 30 minutes.

Chicken au Jus des Pommes

4 Servings

4 chicken breasts, skinned
   and halved
4 small apples
1 teaspoon sugar

Salt
2 tablespoons butter
⅔ cup apple juice (you may
   need to add more)

Broil chicken, turning once, until just lightly browned—about 10 minutes.

Meanwhile, peel and core apples and slice thinly. Place half the apple slices in the bottom of a lightly buttered flat baking dish. Place the broiled chicken breasts on top. Add remaining apple slices; sprinkle with 1 teaspoon sugar and salt to taste. Dot with butter.

Pour apple juice over all, and bake in 375° oven for 1 hour. Check after 30 minutes to see if more apple juice should be added.

Chicken Breasts Eden

4 Servings

3 chicken breasts, skinned and halved
1 package (3 ounces) dried beef
1 can cream of chicken soup

2 cups hot, cooked rice
1 cup commercial sour cream
1 package (3 ounces) cream cheese

Place chicken breasts in a single layer in a baking pan. Separate slices of dried beef, and place over chicken; then spoon soup (undiluted) over meats, and cover pan with foil. Bake in 325° oven for 1 hour; then uncover, and bake an additional 20 minutes or until chicken is tender.

While chicken is baking, cook rice.

Remove chicken from pan when done, and keep warm. Pour pan juices into a small saucepan; add sour cream and cream cheese. Heat slowly, stirring constantly, until cheese melts and sauce is hot.

Spoon rice onto a heated serving platter, and arrange chicken on top. Pour part of the sauce over the chicken, and serve the rest separately.

Sidney's Baked Chicken

4 Servings

4 chicken breasts, skinned
   and halved
4 teaspoons butter
Salt
4 thin slices lemon

2 tablespoons dry sherry
½ cup heavy cream
4 slices mild American
   cheese

Put the chicken breasts in a shallow roasting pan. Dot each piece with ½ teaspoon butter, sprinkle with salt, and bake in 350° oven for 30 minutes.

Meanwhile, cut each lemon slice in half, so that you have a thin *half*-slice for each breast. After 30 minutes cooking time, remove chicken from oven, and place half a lemon slice on each piece of chicken.

Mix the sherry and cream together, and pour over chicken. Return to 350° oven, and cook for 30 minutes, or until chicken is tender.

Remove chicken from oven, and discard lemon slices. Cut 4 thin slices of mild American cheese in half, and place a slice on each piece of chicken. Return to oven, and bake until cheese melts, about 10 minutes.

Chicken Dreams

4 Servings

4 chicken breasts, cut in
   half, skinned, and boned
Salt

1 package (8 ounces) cream
   cheese
10 teaspoons butter

Spread prepared chicken breasts on a large wooden chopping board. Remove odd bits of fat, and pound chicken flat with a mallet. Sprinkle lightly with salt.

Form cream cheese into 8 small balls, about the size of a prune or walnut. Put 1 cream cheese ball and 1 teaspoon butter inside each chicken breast half. Fold the breast around the cream cheese and butter to make a roll, also folding over ends. Secure with toothpicks. Dot with remaining butter.

Broil on a rack, about 8 inches from flame, with a drip pan underneath. Broil for about 30 minutes, turning once or twice. Remove from broiler, discard toothpicks, and serve.

Chicken Tai-Pan

4 Servings

4 chicken breasts, cut in half, skinned, and boned	1½ cups clear chicken broth
Salt	2 teaspoons cornstarch
1 cup cooked rice	1 can (11 ounces) mandarin-orange segments, drained
1 tablespoon butter, melted	

Spread and flatten out the chicken breasts (that have been cut in half and boned) on a large chopping board. Sprinkle the insides lightly with salt.

In a mixing bowl, combine the cooked rice and melted butter, then spoon about 2 to 3 tablespoons of this mixture into each chicken breast. Fold the edges of the chicken breast over the rice stuffing, and secure with toothpicks.

Broil the chicken rolls about 8 inches from the broiler flame, just until they are nicely golden brown. Turn once during broiling time. Remove from broiler.

Put the chicken broth in a large skillet, and heat to boiling point. Add the broiled chicken rolls; reduce heat, and simmer for about 20 minutes, or until chicken is tender. Remove chicken, and keep warm.

Add a little water to the cornstarch to make a paste, then stir into hot chicken broth. Stir constantly until sauce thickens. Stir in drained mandarin-orange segments. Return chicken rolls to sauce mixture for a few minutes, basting several times, before serving.

Poulet en Aspic Rose

2 to 3 Servings, if main luncheon dish
4 to 6 Servings, if served as a salad on a buffet table

4 chicken drumsticks	1½ tablespoon unflavored gelatin
4 chicken thighs	½ cup cold water
1 can beef consommé	1 can (7¼ ounces) tiny Belgian carrots, drained
1 can tomato soup	1 can (7¼ ounces) tiny young peas, drained
3 eggs, hard-cooked	
½ avocado, sliced thinly	

After removing the skin, put chicken pieces in a large saucepan, add soups (undiluted), and bring to a boil. Cover, and simmer for 45 minutes, or until meat is about to fall off the bones. When chicken is done, remove from broth, and set aside to cool slightly.

While chicken is cooking, hard cook eggs, peel, cool and slice. Peel and slice avocado.

Soften gelatin in ½ cup cold water for 5 minutes, then add to hot broth, stirring until dissolved. Pour a thin layer of this aspic into a 6-cup mold that has been rinsed in cold water. Chill.

When chicken is cool enough to handle, take meat off bones, and cut into small pieces. When aspic has stiffened somewhat and clings to the mold, arrange chicken pieces, vegetables, sliced egg, and avocado slices in layers on aspic. Fill mold with remaining aspic. Chill until firm. Serve with our mayonnaise, page 197.

Mormi's Creamed Chicken

2 to 3 Servings

4 pieces of chicken thighs or breasts	2 cups water
	1 can chicken noodle soup

Wash chicken, and remove skin. Place chicken pieces and skin in a large saucepan with a lid, and cover wih 2 cups of water. Bring to a boil with the lid slightly off so that the steam can escape. When the water is boiling, reduce heat to simmer, and cook for 30 minutes, or until the chicken is tender.

While chicken is simmering, take 1 can chicken noodle soup (undiluted), and pour into blender. Blend for 40 seconds.

When chicken is done, remove from heat, and discard skin. Put chicken pieces in a buttered baking dish.

Mix a tablespoon or two of the chicken stock with the chicken noodle soup that has been blended. Pour mixture over cooked chicken, and pop into 375° oven for 20 minutes.

Scalloped Chicken and Eggs

4 Servings

3 tablespoons butter
1½ cups breadcrumbs
2 cups cooked chicken, diced

1 cup milk
2 eggs, well beaten
Salt

Melt 2 tablespoons butter in the top of a double boiler; add 1 cup of the breadcrumbs, and mix well. Line a medium-size baking dish with this mixture. Pack down firmly in baking dish. Cover with the chicken.

Heat 1 tablespoon butter with 1 cup milk in the top of a double boiler, and when hot (not boiling) stir in remaining ½ cup breadcrumbs. Stir in well-beaten eggs a little at a time, add salt to taste, and mix thoroughly.

Pour mixture over chicken. Top with a sprinkling of breadcrumbs. Bake in 375° oven for 30 minutes.

Normandy Chicken Casserole

4 Servings

1 can cream of chicken soup
⅓ cup milk
1 cup cooked chicken, diced
1 cup noodles, cooked

1 cup green beans, cooked
Salt
Breadcrumbs
1 tablespoon butter

In a mixing bowl, blend soup with the milk. Add the cubed chicken, and the cooked noodles and green beans. Mix well, and add salt to taste. Spoon into a 1½-quart casserole, top with breadcrumbs, and dot with butter. Bake in 400° oven for 25 minutes.

Chicken Noodle Casserole

4 to 6 Servings

1 box (8 ounces) medium-size noodles
1 package (8 ounces) cream cheese
1 cup non-fat creamed cottage cheese
1 cup commercial sour cream
Salt
2 cups cooked chicken, diced
¼ cup grated Parmesan cheese

Cook noodles according to directions on box. When done, drain, and set aside.

In a large mixing bowl, soften cream cheese. When soft, add cottage cheese, sour cream, and salt to taste. Mix well. Add cooked noodles, and combine thoroughly but gently.

Butter a 2-quart casserole. Arrange a layer of noodles on the bottom, then a layer of cooked chicken, and continue alternating noodles and chicken until all are used. Top with ¼ cup grated Parmesan cheese. Bake in 350° oven for 1 hour. Do not bake longer, as this dish will become too hard.

Chicken Roulade

6 Servings

6 tablespoons butter
¾ cup *sifted* flour
3½ cups milk
Salt

4 eggs, separated
2 cups cooked chicken,
   finely diced

Butter a 15 x 10 x 1-inch jelly-roll pan, then line with waxed paper. Butter waxed paper, and lightly dust with flour.

Melt butter in the top of a double boiler; stir in ¾ cup of flour and mix well. Add 3 cups of the milk, and stir constantly until mixture becomes very thick. Add salt to taste. When mixture has thickened, *remove 1 cup and set aside for later use.*

Beat egg whites until they are stiff. In a separate bowl, beat egg yolks until they are light and lemon-colored. Stir 1 tablespoon at a time into the 2 cups of white-sauce mixture in the double boiler. Blend very well. Pour into a large mixing bowl.

Carefully fold in stiff egg whites, until no streaks remain. Spread evenly on jelly-roll pan, and bake this omelet mixture in 325° oven for 1 hour.

While this is baking, put the cup of white sauce that had been set aside into the top of a double boiler. Add remaining ½ cup milk and diced chicken. Keep on low heat.

When omelet is done, remove from pan by loosening around edges with a spatula or knife. Cover with waxed paper or foil, then place a large cookie sheet on top, and quickly turn over. Lift pan off and peel off waxed paper. Spoon chicken mixture in a layer over omelet, then roll up like a jelly roll. Cut into 6 slices with a sharp knife. Serve immediately.

Chicken Épinard

6 Servings

2 packages frozen chopped
   spinach
2 tablespoons butter
2 tablespoons flour
1 cup chicken broth
½ cup milk

Salt
16 thin slices left-over cooked
   chicken
2 tablespoons grated
   Parmesan cheese

Cook the frozen chopped spinach until just thawed, following directions on the package. Drain very well.

Melt 2 tablespoons butter in the top of a double boiler. When melted, stir in 2 tablespoons flour, and blend well. Add chicken broth, milk, and salt to taste. Stir constantly until mixture begins to thicken.

Spread spinach on the bottom of a baking dish. Pour half of the sauce over this. Arrange left-over chicken slices on the spinach and cover with remaining sauce. Sprinkle grated Parmesan cheese on top. Bake in 425° oven for 15 or 20 minutes, until lightly browned.

Chicken-and-Cheese Strata

6 Servings

12 slices day-old bread
½ cup our mayonnaise
   (page 197)
2 cups cooked chicken,
   finely minced

6 slices mild American
   cheese
6 eggs, beaten
2¼ cups milk
Salt

Trim the crusts from the bread slices. Arrange 6 slices in the bottom of a flat 12 x 7 x 2-inch baking dish. Spread each slice of bread with mayonnaise, then cover these with a layer of finely minced chicken. Put a slice of cheese on top of each bread slice, then top with the 6 remaining pieces of bread.

Beat the eggs thoroughly, add the milk, and salt to taste. Pour this mixture over the sandwiches in the baking dish, and refrigerate for 1 hour.

Then bake in a 325° oven for 1 hour. Serve immediately.

Chicken Livers en Brochette

3 Servings

1 pound chicken livers
3 to 4 tablespoons butter,
  melted

1 cup breadcrumbs

Wash and dry chicken livers; remove any extra bits of fat. Dip livers in the melted butter, and then coat with breadcrumbs.

Thread the livers on 3 eight-inch skewers. Place on buttered broiler rack, and broil 6 inches from heat for about 3 minutes on each side, or until tender.

Russian Chicken Livers

3 Servings

1 pound chicken livers
1 cup commercial sour
  cream

½ cup clear chicken broth
Salt

Broil chicken livers just until they have lost their pinkness —do *not* overcook.

Meanwhile, combine sour cream and chicken broth in a saucepan, and heat slowly until the mixture is bubbly. Add broiled livers to the sauce. Season with salt to taste—but remember, chicken broth itself is salty. Cover, and cook over low heat for 5 minutes. Serve on rice or toast, or with boiled new potatoes.

Chicken Livers Supreme

4 Servings

2 tablespoons butter	2 whole eggs
2 tablespoons flour	2 egg yolks
1 cup milk	6 tablespoons heavy cream
Salt	1 tablespoon cognac
½ pound chicken livers	1 can cream of celery soup

Set oven at 350°

Melt butter in the top of a double boiler. When melted, stir in flour and mix well. Add milk, salt to taste, and stir constantly until sauce is smooth and begins to thicken. Set aside to cool slightly, but do not refrigerate. Sir sauce occasionally while it is cooling.

Put chicken livers, whole eggs, and egg yolks in a blender, and blend for 1 minute. Add the cooled sauce, cream, and cognac, and blend for 15 seconds.

Pour mixture into a 1-quart baking dish, and set baking dish in a pan of hot water. Bake in preheated 350° oven for 30 minutes, or until set. Unmold onto a warm platter.

Serve with this quick celery sauce: About 10 minutes before chicken livers are done, put the contents of one can of cream of celery soup (undiluted) in a blender. Blend until soup is smooth and has a saucelike consistency—about 15 seconds. Pour into saucepan, and heat over low flame until sauce is hot.

Sherried Chicken Livers

3 Servings

1 pound chicken livers   Butter
2 to 3 tablespoons sherry

Put chicken livers in a sieve, and rinse with cold water. Drain on paper towels, and remove odd bits of fat. Arrange chicken livers on broiling rack, and broil approximately 5 minutes on each side. When turning the livers, sprinkle with sherry and dot with butter. Serve immediately.

Chicken Liver and Rice Casserole

4 Servings

1 package frozen chopped   2 tablespoons Burgundy
  spinach   wine
1⅓ cups packaged, pre-   1 cup grated Parmesan
  cooked rice   cheese
½ pound chicken livers   Salt
2 tablespoons butter

Thaw spinach, and drain.
Cook the rice according to directions on box.
Wash, dry, and clean the chicken livers, cutting off any bits of fat. Broil until barely done, then cut into small pieces.

Combine the spinach, rice, chicken livers, butter, wine, cheese, and salt to taste. Mix well. Spoon into a 1½-quart casserole, and bake, covered, in 350° oven for 25 minutes.

Cornish Hen in a Package

Allow one-half Rock Cornish hen per person. (If the hens are very small, use a whole hen per person and adjust recipe ingredients.)

Salt	2 tablespoons butter for each
1 teaspoon breadcrumbs for each half hen	half hen

Defrost, wash, and split each hen in half. Dry with paper towels. Sprinkle each half with salt to taste and breadcrumbs. Dot each half on skin side with 2 tablespoons butter.

Preheat oven to 425°.

Put each half hen into a heavy brown paper bag. Fold open end of each bag, and seal with cellophane tape, or fasten with paper clips. Put bags on a large cookie sheet, and place in oven. Turn oven down to 375°, and bake for a good 45 minutes. If package begins to scorch, cover with a sheet of foil.

Cut open paper bags directly after removing from oven, and serve hens immediately. If left to stand in the bags, they will become soggy.

Lean Duck Rôti

3 to 4 Servings

1 duckling, about 4 pounds
Salt
2 cups orange juice

Dash of Brandy
2 oranges, sliced, for garnish

Wash duckling, and rub with salt. Prick the skin to allow fat to drain. Broil *on a spit* in broiler or rotisserie for 1½ to 2 hours, or 25 to 30 minutes per pound. When done, let duckling cool until it can be handled.

With poultry shears, cut duck into small pieces. Separate the legs from the thighs and the wings from the breast. Snip off wing-tips, and discard; remove backbone. Remove skin and fat from all pieces.

Put cut-up pieces of duck into a shallow baking pan. Cover with orange juice and brandy, and reheat in 350° oven for about 15 minutes, or until duckling and juices are hot. Place on a warm platter, and surround with orange slices for garnish. Serve sauce separately.

Turkey in Champagne

*12 to 15 Servings, with
meat left over for another meal*

12-to 15-pound turkey
Salt
Butter

1 cup beef consommé
1 pint (split) champagne

Wash the turkey, and rub inside and out with salt. (Use salt sparingly, as consómmé will also add salt.) Close the turkey openings with poultry pins and string. Tie legs together, and twist wings so tips are flat against the turkey back. Rub turkey with butter, and place breast-side-up in a large open roasting pan.

Roast in 425° oven for 30 minutes; then pour consommé over bird. Reduce oven to 235°, and roast for 1 hour.

After 1 hour and 30 minutes' roasting time, pour champagne over turkey. Continue roasting for 3½ hours for a 12-pound turkey—or 4 hours for a 15-pound turkey. Baste frequently.

You will note that this recipe does not call for turkey stuffing, which, because of the spices, most ulcer patients have trouble digesting. However, for the rest of the family, this turkey is also delicious with stuffing.

Turkey Divan

4 Servings

Traditionally, Turkey Divan is made with broccoli. However, since broccoli is a marginal vegetable for an ulcer patient, we've substituted asparagus.

1 package frozen asparagus spears	4 large thin slices cooked white meat of turkey
4 slices white bread	Salt
butter	½ cup grated mild American cheese
1 cup commercial sour cream	

Cook asparagus according to directions on package, and drain well.

Toast bread slices, then butter lightly. Cover the bottom of a large flat baking dish with the buttered toast. Put a slice of turkey over each piece of toast, sprinkle with salt, and top with asparagus spears. Spoon sour cream in ribbons over asparagus. Sprinkle with grated cheese. Bake in 400° oven for 20 minutes, or until cheese melts.

Fish

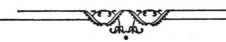

Fish is an excellent food in terms of both nutrition and taste. Even though ulcer patients must not eat shellfish, there is still such a variety of fish available that seafood can be served at least once a week.

We are not going to tell you how to broil, steam, or bake fish, but for the patient just going on to solid foods, here is a tip when boiling fish: start with *cold* water, and add a reasonable amount of salt and a drop of lemon juice. You may even add a bay leaf, as long as this is put in a little pouch that can be removed when the fish is done. Bring water to a boil, and immediately reduce to simmer. Simmer fillets 6 minutes per pound; whole fish 8 minutes per pound. *Simmer* is the operative word.

Buy only very fresh fish from a reputable fishery; or quick-frozen fish, marketed under a well-known label and sold in a store with proper storage facilities. Remember that fish does not require long cooking.

A high-protein, low-calorie fish course can be followed by a fairly splendid dessert.

Baked Halibut au Gratin

2 Servings

2 pounds halibut steak
1 teaspoon salt
4 tablespoons butter

½ cup breadcrumbs
¼ cup grated Parmesan
   cheese

Put the halibut in a buttered baking dish, sprinkle with salt, and dot with 2 tablespoons of butter. Bake in 350° oven for 15 minutes. Cover with mixture of breadcrumbs and grated cheese, dot with remaining butter, and bake an additional 15 minutes or until the crumbs are browned and the fish flaky.

Snowy Halibut Steaks

4 Servings

1 to 2 celery stalks, scraped
   and thinly sliced
4 halibut steaks, cut ¾-inch
   thick

1 tablespoon lemon juice
½ teaspoon salt
¼ cup sour cream

Place celery in a shallow baking dish with lid, and put halibut steaks on top. Brush steaks with lemon juice, sprinkle with salt, and cover. Bake in 400° oven for 20 minutes, then uncover.

Spread each steak with 1 tablespoon of the sour cream. Bake 10 minutes longer, until fish flakes easily.

Paper-Baked Pompano

---

4 Servings

Bluefish or striped bass can also be cooked this way.

2 to 3 pounds of Pompano   1 tablespoon lemon juice
Salt to taste   3 tablespoons butter

Sprinkle fish with a little salt and lemon juice, then dot with butter.

Take a heavy brown paper bag (the bag should be large enough to wrap around the fish) and rub the inside with butter. Place the fish inside the bag, and fold the edges of the bag *securely;* fasten with paper clips or cellophane tape.

Put in a baking dish, and bake in 350° oven for 45 minutes. If the package begins to scorch, cover with a sheet of foil. Serve the fish immediately after unwrapping.

Filets of Sole Vin Blanc Sec

---

2 Servings

1½ pounds fillets of sole   Butter
1 cup dry white wine   2 egg yolks
Salt   ½ cup heavy cream

Arrange the fillets in a shallow baking dish. Add white wine; sprinkle the fillets with salt to taste, and dot generously with butter. Bake in 350° oven for 20 minutes, or until fish is cooked but still firm. (If the fillets are small, you may need less time). Remove from oven.

Drain liquid that is in the baking dish into a small sauce-pan. Simmer it down to about 1 cup. Mix egg yolks with cream, and stir mixture carefully into the reduced fish stock. Pour sauce over the fish, and pop briefly under a hot broiler.

Sole with Soufflé Sauce

2 to 3 Servings

2 pounds fillets of sole
Salt
2 egg whites

½ cup our mayonnaise
(page 197)

Sprinkle fish with salt to taste, and arrange in a lightly buttered shallow baking pan. Broil, with the fish about 4 to 6 inches from the flame, for 10 to 15 minutes. Remove pan from broiler, but leave broiler on.

Beat egg whites until stiff but not dry, then fold into ½ cup of mayonnaise. Spread this sauce over the top of the fish, and return to broiler for 3 minutes, or until sauce is puffy and lightly browned.

Fish Turbans

3 Servings

1 package frozen creamed
spinach
¾ pound fillets of sole or
flounder

Lemon juice
2 tablespoons butter, melted
Salt
1 egg, beaten

Cook spinach according to directions on package.

Sprinkle fish with lemon juice, and cut into strips, about 3 to 4 strips per fillet.

Butter sides of 3 custard cups with melted butter mixed with a little salt, and put fillet strips around the sides. Brush with rest of butter.

Mix creamed spinach with egg, and fill center of custard cups. Bake in 375° oven for about 30 minutes, until fish is done and center is set. Unmold on hot plates.

Stuffed Fish Rolls

3 to 4 Servings

1 cup breadcrumbs
4 tablespoons butter, melted

1½ pounds fillets of sole or flounder
Salt

Mix breadcrumbs with 3 tablespoons melted butter.

Cut fish fillets into strips about 5 inches long, and sprinkle with a little salt. Coat fillets with breadcrumb mixture, roll, and fasten with toothpicks.

Place fish rolls in a buttered baking dish, brush with remaining tablespoon of butter, and bake in 350° oven for 25 minutes.

Creamed Fillets

2 Servings

1 pound fish fillets
½ teaspoon salt
Breadcrumbs

4 teaspoons butter
About ¾ cup cream

Sprinkle fish with salt. Place fillets close together in a shallow buttered baking dish; sprinkle with breadcrumbs, and dot with butter. Add cream until fish is half covered. Bake in 350° oven for about 30 minutes.

Boneless Red Snapper

2 Servings

1 red snapper (about 2 pounds)
Boiling salted water

½ cup olive oil
Juice of 1 lemon
Salt

Wrap cleaned fish in cheesecloth and place in a large skillet. Cover fish with boiling salted water, and simmer gently for about 15 minutes, or until done. Carefully lift fish onto oven-proof platter, and let cool. Do not refrigerate.

When cool, remove cheesecloth and slice fish open to remove bones. Mix oil, lemon juice, and a dash of salt, and pour mixture over the fish.

Preheat broiler. Put the fish on its platter in the broiler, but not too close to flame, and brown lightly. Serve at once.

Poached Salmon Steaks

4 Servings

1 large lemon, cut in 6 slices	4 salmon steaks (each 1-inch thick)
½ teaspoon salt	Our Hollandaise Sauce (page 198)

Half fill a heavy skillet (about 11 inches) with water, add 2 to 3 lemon slices and salt. Heat just to boiling. Put salmon steaks in pan and cover. Simmer 15 minutes, until fish flakes easily. Drain, and serve on heated platter with our Hollandaise and remaining lemon slices for garnish.

Poached Salmon with Lemon Butter

4 Servings

1 cup dry white wine	Salt
2 cups water	4 salmon steaks
1 stalk celery, scraped and finely minced	4 tablespoons butter, melted
	4 tablespoons lemon juice

In a large skillet bring wine, water, celery, and a dash of salt to a boil. Reduce heat; simmer, covered, for 15 minutes.

Meanwhile, rinse salmon steaks in cold water, and drain. Place salmon in wine mixture, adding water if needed, so liquid just covers salmon. Return to boil, reduce heat, and simmer, covered, for 15 minutes, or until the fish flakes easily when tested with a fork.

Remove salmon from skillet with a wide slotted spatula, and drain. Place on heated serving platter. Combine melted butter and lemon juice. Drizzle mixture over salmon. Garnish with lemon slices.

Instant Hot Salmon

2 Servings

1 can (7¾ ounces) salmon
 in water pack
Lemon juice

4 tablespoons commercial
 sour cream
3 tablespoons milk

Drain salmon and remove any skin. Divide salmon between 2 individual baking ramekins (4½ inches in diameter).

Sprinkle a few drops of lemon juice on the salmon. Thin the sour cream with the milk, and spoon over fish.

Put ramekins in broiler, not too close to heat, and broil until fish is bubbly and browned—for about 8 to 10 minutes.

Salmon and Rice Loaf

6 Servings

1 can (16 ounces) salmon
2 eggs
2 cups cooked rice
2 tablespoons butter, melted

1 stalk celery, finely chopped
2 teaspoons lemon juice
¼ cup water
Salt

Break the salmon into chunks, drain, remove dark skin and bones.

Beat eggs in a large mixing bowl, add salmon and cooked rice. Mix in all other ingredients, and add salt to taste. Blend thoroughly, and pack into a lightly buttered loaf pan. Bake in 375° oven for 40 minutes, or until firm to touch in the middle.

Salmon Soufflé

4 Servings

2 cans (7¾ ounces each)
   salmon in water pack
¼ teaspoon salt
2 tablespoons lemon juice

½ cup milk
½ cup breadcrumbs
3 eggs, separated

Drain the fish and separate into flakes, being sure all bones and skin are removed. Mix fish with salt and lemon juice.

Put the milk and breadcrumbs into the top of a double boiler, and heat until well blended.

Beat the egg yolks well, then beat the egg whites until stiff.

Add the fish to the milk and breadcrumb mixture, then add the egg yolks, but do not overheat. Fold the egg whites into the mixture.

Now spoon the mixture into a buttered baking dish. Set the dish in a pan of hot water, and bake in a 350° oven for 30 minutes, or until firm.

This is particularly good when served with our Hollandaise Sauce, page 198.

Fish Puff

3 to 4 Servings

This recipe can be served as a main course at lunch, or as an appetizer.

1 can (16 ounces) carrots, drained
3 eggs, separated

1 can (7 ounces) tuna in water pack
2 tablespoons lemon juice
Salt

Put carrots in blender and purée, or mash through a sieve. Beat egg yolks well, and add to carrot purée.

Drain the fish, and carefully fold into carrot mixture, adding lemon juice and a dash of salt. Beat egg whites until stiff and fold into mixture.

Bake in medium-size casserole in 350° oven for 30 minutes, until dish is golden brown on top. Serve at once, possibly with Sauce Verte, page 198, or tomato soup diluted with a little milk and heated as sauce.

Tuna Italiano

4 Servings

2 cans (7 ounces each) tuna in water pack
1 cup grated Parmesan cheese
1 egg

½ cup milk
1 tablespoon butter, melted
1 carrot, grated
3 tablespoons breadcrumbs
Salt

Drain tuna and put in a bowl. Add grated Parmesan cheese, and combine well.

Put egg, milk, and melted butter in a blender, and blend for a few seconds. Pour into tuna-cheese mixture. Add grated carrot, 1 tablespoon breadcrumbs, and a dash of salt. Mix well, and pack into a buttered loaf pan. Sprinkle remaining 2 tablespoons breadcrumbs on top. Bake in 375° oven for 45 minutes.

Potatoes

Potatoes supply bulk—which the ulcer patient needs to help regulate elimination—and the mineral content produces an alkaline reaction. The stomach that has been ulcerated needs all the help it can get in maintaining a healthy acid-alkaline balance, so keep the portions small, but serve potatoes. They are also a good source of the B vitamins, vitamin C, iron, and, of course, carbohydrates for energy.

A potato, boiled or baked, contains approximately 100 calories—about the same number as one cup of orange juice. It is what you add to the potato, or what you serve with it, that makes it fattening. So, for proper weight control, and to ensure easy digestion, serve a sophisticated potato recipe with a plain meat dish. Our potato cheese soufflé is an excellent companion for a simple steak or ground-beef dinner. Danish new potatoes can accompany a more complicated meat dish.

Pare potatoes as thinly as possible. The maximum amount of food value is near the skin, which the ulcer patient must never eat.

Hostess Potatoes

6 Servings

12 medium-small, firm
  potatoes
½ cup butter, melted

1 cup grated Parmesan
  cheese
Salt

Boil potatoes, and peel them. While still warm, roll them in melted butter and then in cheese mixed with salt. Place on well-buttered baking sheet and bake in preheated 400° oven for about 15 minutes. Turn potatoes once, to crust on both sides.

Dutch Potatoes

4 to 6 Servings

6 medium potatoes
¾ to 1 cup breadcrumbs
1 to 1½ cups milk

4 to 5 tablespoons butter
Salt

Boil potatoes in lightly salted water for 15 minutes. Drain. When cool enough to handle, peel and slice.

Cover the bottom of a buttered baking dish with breadcrumbs mixed with bits of butter. Add a layer of sliced potatoes, and sprinkle with salt. Alternate crumbs (dotted with butter) and lightly salted potato slices until all are used. Pour milk over all, and bake in 350° oven for 35 to 45 minutes.

Scalloped Potatoes Milky Way

4 to 6 Servings

6 medium potatoes
2 tablespoons flour
Salt

4 to 5 tablespoons butter
Milk

Scrub potatoes, peel, and cut into thin slices. Place in buttered baking dish in 3 layers, about 1-inch deep in all, sprinkling each layer with a bit of flour and salt, and dotting with butter. Add milk, until it can be seen between slices of potatoes.

Cover, and bake in 350° oven for 45 minutes. Remove cover, and let potatoes brown for 15 minutes. They are done if tender when pierced with a fork.

Danish New Potatoes

4 Servings

12 small new potatoes

4 tablespoons granulated sugar or brown sugar

Boil small, firm new potatoes with the skins on. Normal cooking time is about 30 minutes. Peel potatoes when done and cool enough to handle.

Just before serving, take a teflon frying pan, and spread 4 tablespoons of sugar in it. Heat over low flame until sugar begins to bubble, then quickly turn the potatoes into the melted sugar. Shake pan over low heat for a few minutes. A delicious glaze will form around the potatoes.

The last step of this recipe *must* be done just prior to eating, as sugar burns easily.

New Potatoes and Beans, French Style

6 Servings

12 small new potatoes	1 package frozen string
Salt	beans, French style
3 tablespoons butter	1½ tablespoons cornstarch
	1 tablespoon water

Wash and peel potatoes. Pour one inch of water into a large pan that has a cover, add salt to taste, and bring to a boil. Add potatoes and butter; cover, and cook for 20 minutes over low heat.

Add frozen string beans, and cook until beans are tender, following directions for cooking time on package. Remove potatoes and beans from pan, and reserve the liquid.

Mix cornstarch and 1 tablespoon water into a smooth paste. Add to reserved liquid and cook over low heat for 1 minute, stirring constantly, until sauce is transparent and just slightly thick. Return vegetables to sauce, and warm over low heat for 1 minute.

Potatoes Killarney

8 Servings

4 large baking potatoes	Salt
1 package frozen creamed	3 slices mild American
spinach	cheese
1 egg yolk	

Bake potatoes. Heat spinach according to package directions.

After potatoes are baked, cut in half and scoop out insides, leaving shells intact. Blend potatoes with egg yolk, salt to taste, and spinach until smooth. Refill shells with potato-spinach mixture, topping high. Cut cheese into small strips, and place crosswise on top. Put under broiler until cheese is melted.

Potato Charlotte

4 Servings

2 slices stale white bread of a fine texture
Milk, enough for soaking bread
3 cups coarsely grated raw potatoes (about 3 large potatoes)

2 eggs, beaten
Salt
1 cup grated mild American cheese

Set oven at 350°.

Place bread in a shallow bowl or pan, and add enough milk so that both slices will soak thoroughly.

Mix grated potatoes, beaten eggs, salt to taste, and cheese in a medium-size bowl.

Squeeze most of the milk from the bread slices, and add bread to potato mixture. Mix very well. Turn into a buttered 1-quart casserole, and bake in preheated oven for 1 hour. Serve immediately.

Potato Cheese Soufflé

4 Servings

2 cups hot mashed potatoes
4 eggs, separated
2 tablespoons butter

½ cup grated Parmesan
   cheese
½ cup milk
Salt

Make mashed potatoes in your usual way, or use dehydrated mashed potatoes.

Separate eggs, and mix potatoes and lightly beaten egg yolks with the butter, grated cheese, milk, and salt to taste. Whip until light and fluffy.

Beat egg whites until stiff but not dry; fold into potato mixture. Mix lightly, and turn into a buttered soufflé dish. Bake in 350° oven for 20 minutes. Serve at once.

Norwegian Potato Pudding

4 Servings

2 cups hot dehydrated
   mashed potatoes
2 eggs, separated
½ cup cream

Salt
¼ cup breadcrumbs
1 tablespoon butter

Prepare mashed potatoes according to directions on box.

Beat egg yolks, and stir into mashed potatoes. Add cream and salt to taste, mixing well.

Beat egg whites until stiff but not dry, and fold into mixture. Turn into a lightly buttered casserole, and top with breadcrumbs. Dot with butter. Bake in 350° oven for 30 minutes. Serve immediately.

Golden Mashed Potatoes

4 Servings

4 meduim-size carrots
2 cups hot dehydrated
   mashed potatoes

Salt to taste

Wash and scrape carrots, and cook until very soft. When done and cool enough to handle, cut into small pieces, and put in a blender. Blend until carrots are puréed.

Meanwhile, make mashed potatoes according to directions on box. Add potatoes to carrots in blender. Blend until potatoes and carrots are smooth and a golden color. Add salt to taste. Warm in a small saucepan over very low heat.

This is an especially good recipe for anyone just going onto a solid-food ulcer diet.

Sweet Potato de Luxe

4 Servings

3 large sweet potatoes
2 eggs, separated
2 tablespoons butter
½ cup cream

1½ tablespoons brown
  sugar
1 teaspoon grated orange
  rind
Salt

Cook potatoes in boiling salted water for 30 minutes, or until tender. When cool enough to handle, peel and mash.

Separate the eggs. Beat yolks, then add butter, cream, brown sugar, orange rind, and salt to taste. Continue beating until mixture is fluffy. Fold into mashed potatoes.

Beat egg whites until they stand in firm peaks, then carefully fold into potato mixture. Turn into a 1-quart casserole, and bake in 325° oven for 1 hour.

Sweet Potato Pudding

4 Servings

2 cups sweet potatoes (about
  3 large sweet potatoes)
1 cup brown sugar
½ cup light corn syrup

1 cup milk
2 eggs, lightly beaten
2 tablespoons butter, melted
Salt

Set oven at 350°.

Peel potatoes and grate coarsely.

Mix all ingredients in a large bowl until thoroughly blended. Pour into a buttered long, glass baking dish, about 12 x 8 x 2 inches, and bake in preheated oven for 1 hour.

This sweet potato pudding is wonderful with plain roast chicken or lean broiled lamb chops.

Apple-Yam Dandy

6 Servings

6 medium-size yams or sweet
    potatoes
1½ cups peeled apple slices
½ cup brown sugar, firmly
    packed

Salt
4 tablespoons butter

Wash and cook potatoes in boiling water until they can be pierced with a fork. They should be just tender but not over-cooked. Drain; when cool enough to handle, peel and cut into slices about ¼-inch thick.

Butter a 2-quart casserole, and arrange half of the sweet potatoes on the bottom. Cover with half of the apple slices. Sprinkle this layer with ¼ cup brown sugar, a bit of salt, and dot with 2 tablespoons butter. Now add the rest of the sweet potatoes, and then finish off with a layer of the remaining apple slices. Sprinkle the top with salt, and dot with the final 2 tablespoons butter. Bake in 350° oven for 45 minutes.

Sherried Sweet Potatoes

4 Servings

2 medium-size sweet potatoes
   or yams
8 tablespoons sherry
8 tablespoons pineapple
   juice

Salt
4 tablespoons brown sugar
4 tablespoons butter

Wash and cook potatoes in boiling water until tender when pierced with a fork. Drain and let cool. When cool enough to handle, peel, and cut potatoes into 1-inch slices. Arrange in a flat, buttered baking dish. The slices should not overlap.

Mix sherry, pineapple juice, and salt to taste in a small saucepan, and bring to a boil. Pour over potatoes, and bake, in 350° oven for 15 minutes.

Remove from oven, sprinkle brown sugar on top, dot with butter, and put under preheated broiler until sugar melts and browns potatoes slightly. When serving, spoon sauce over potatoes.

Harvest Casserole

4 Servings

1½ to 2 pounds sweet
   potatoes or yams, enough
   to make 3 cups mashed
   potatoes
4 tablespoons butter, melted
3 tablespoons brown sugar

1 tablespoon grated orange
   rind
½ cup orange juice
Salt
6 to 8 marshmallows

Wash and cook potatoes in boiling water until tender when pierced with a fork. Drain; when cool enough to handle, peel and mash potatoes.

Preheat oven to 375°. Combine all ingredients except marshmallows. Mix lightly but very well, and turn into a 1-quart buttered casserole. Bake for 30 minutes. Top with marshallows and place under broiler until marshmallows start to melt and turn golden brown.

Vegetables

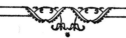

Ulcer sufferers often complain that if they must adhere strictly to the permitted diet, they are very limited in their choice of vegetables. This is not necessarily so. Twenty-nine recipes for vegetables dishes appear in this book, and we are sure you will be pleasantly surprised at the imaginative combinations that are perfectly acceptable for sensitive stomachs.

Admittedly, cabbage, cauliflower, corn, sauerkraut, brussels sprouts, onion, lima beans, dried peas and dried beans, old beets, and all raw vegetables (radishes, cucumbers, green peppers, uncooked carrots) are not allowed. Raw vegetables have a cell wall of inert carbohydrate-cellulose that the troubled stomach simply cannot break down easily.

Peas and broccoli tips are controversial for the ulcer patient. We are, however, suggesting a few recipes featuring these popular vegetables, because so many diet lists include them for those who are ready for a nearly normal selection of foods. Buy only young and unwilted fresh vegetables. If these are not available, frozen or canned vegetables are always preferable to old and large fresh vegetables.

The method of preparing vegetables for cooking is extremely important. Carrots, for example, must be carefully scraped; strings should be removed from string beans; stems removed from fresh spinach. Fresh asparagus must be carefully scrutinized and washed. Be certain that the tips are free of sand, and be ruthless about breaking off the tough stalks. If you don't own an asparagus cooker, lay the asparagus in a large pot in alternate criss-cross layers, with room between each stalk, before adding water and salt. This will insure thorough overall cooking.

Tomato is a perfectly acceptable food for the ulcerated stomach to digest, provided it is cooked and peeled. (When left unpeeled, as in the case of baked stuffed tomatoes, the patient must not eat the outer skin.) To peel a tomato easily, leave it a few minutes in scalding water, or hold under very hot running water at the end of a fork. Dip immediately into very cold water, nick the skin with a sharp knife, and peel.

Vegetables served to the ulcer patient must be well-cooked —but that does not mean *overcooked*. Never use soda in cooking vegetables, as this destroys the vitamin content. Use small amounts of water, lightly salted, and follow our cooking methods.

Incidentally, vegetables baked in a casserole retain the maximum amount of vitamin and mineral content.

Directions for Cooking Artichokes

Put a large pot in the sink, and fill with cold water. When the pot is full, keep the faucet turned on, and plunge artichokes up and down in the water until all earth and sand are removed. Then fill the pot with fresh cold water. Let the artichokes stand in this water, head down, for 30 minutes. Drain the artichokes, trim the stems close, and strip off the outer leaves. With scissors, cut off tough leaf-tops.

Tie a piece of string around each artichoke. Place in a steamer above salted water. Cover tightly, and steam 45 minutes to 1 hour, until the leaves are tender. Cooking time depends, of course, on the size of the artichoke. Drain artichokes, and discard the string.

If you wish to remove the fibrous choke, separate the leaves very carefully, and scoop it out of the "core." A grapefruit spoon comes in handy for doing this, or a small paring knife. You must be deft, otherwise you will detach the outer leaves or scoop out too much of the artichoke heart.

Artichokes Saint Germain

3 to 4 Servings

1 package frozen tiny peas
1½ teaspoons butter
¼ cup heavy cream

Salt
1 can artichoke *bottoms*

Cook peas in saucepan according to directions on package. When done, drain, and put in blender to purée. Return purée to saucepan, and heat over very low heat until the purée is quite dry.

Add butter, cream, and salt to taste. Stir constantly until butter is melted and cream is thoroughly heated.

Meanwhile, heat artichoke bottoms in their liquid over low flame. Drain. Fill artichoke bottoms with purée of peas and serve.

Artichokes à la Sidney

6 Servings

1 package frozen artichoke
   hearts
2 cups sliced cooked carrots

⅓ cup clear chicken broth
1 tablespoon butter
Salt

Cook the artichoke hearts according to directions on package, but shorten cooking time by 2 minutes. Drain them, and put into a medium-size saucepan. Add sliced cooked carrots. Pour in the chicken broth, and cook slowly until the broth has evaporated—about 5 minutes. Add butter and salt to taste. Stir well.

Asparagus with Summer Squash

4 Servings

2 medium-size summer
   squash
12 asparagus spears
2 tablespoons butter
2 tablespoons flour
1 cup light cream

½ cup grated mild
   American cheese
1 tablespoon grated
   Parmesan cheese
Salt

Wash and scrape summer squash; slice in thin rounds. Boil in lightly salted water for 20 minutes. Drain; put into blender, and purée. Return to saucepan, and keep warm.

Meanwhile, wash asparagus, and carefully break off tough part of stalks. Cook asparagus in boiling water for 10 to 15 minutes. Drain, and keep warm.

In the top of a double boiler, melt the butter. When melted, stir in flour. Blend very well, then pour in cream. Stir until mixture is smooth and begins to thicken. Add the grated American cheese and grated Parmesan cheese. Stir very well; add salt to taste.

Put puréed summer squash in serving bowl; arrange asparagus spears on top. Pour sauce mixture over all, and serve.

Scalloped Asparagus and Egg Casserole

4 Servings

1 bunch asparagus
  (about 2 pounds)
3 eggs, hard-cooked
5 tablespoons butter

4 tablespoons flour
2 cups milk
Salt
½ cup breadcrumbs

Wash asparagus, and carefully break off tough part of stems. Cut asparagus into 2-inch pieces, and cook in boiling water about 10 minutes, until just barely tender. Drain.

Slice hard-cooked eggs.

In a medium-size baking dish, put a layer of asparagus, then a layer of sliced egg, alternating until all are used.

Melt 4 tablespoons butter in the top of a double boiler. When melted, stir in flour, and mix well. Add milk, and salt to taste, and stir constantly until sauce thickens. Pour over asparagus and egg layers. Top with breadcrumbs and remaining 1 tablespoon butter. Bake in 375° oven for 30 minutes, or until lightly browned.

Beets à la Crème

6 Servings

2 tablespoons butter
2 tablespoons flour
1 cup clear chicken broth

½ cup heavy cream
Salt
3 cups canned sliced beets

Melt butter in the top of a double boiler. Stir in flour, and blend well. Add chicken broth, and stir until mixture is smooth and begins to thicken. Stir in the cream, and taste for salt (chicken broth usually provides enough salt). Simmer for about 5 minutes, then add the beets, and heat thoroughly.

Orange-Buttered Beets

4 Servings

2 cans (8¾ ounces each)
    shredded beets
¼ cup orange juice
2 tablespoons butter

1 teaspoon cornstarch
1 teaspoon water
Salt

Combine the shredded beets (do not drain), orange juice, and butter in a saucepan. Bring to the boiling point. Reduce heat, and cook for about 5 minutes.

Mix the cornstarch and water together, and add to the beets. Cook over low heat, stirring constantly, just for a few minutes, until the sauce has thickened. Salt to taste.

The Very Best Carrots in the Whole World

6 Servings

1 pound small, young
  carrots
4 tablespoons water
4 tablespoons butter

2 teaspoons sugar
Salt
½ cup orange juice
Orange slices for garnish

Wash and scrape carrots; grate coarsely.

Put water, butter, and grated carrots in a heavy saucepan. Stir in sugar and salt to taste. Cover, and cook for 10 minutes over medium heat, stirring several times.

Stir in orange juice, and cook 5 minutes longer, until carrots are crisply tender. Garnish with orange wedges, if desired, before serving.

Carrots Glazed with Honey and Orange

4 Servings

2 tablespoons orange juice
2 tablespoons honey
2 tablespoons butter

Salt
3½ cups canned sliced
  carrots

Combine the orange juice, honey, butter, and salt to taste in a saucepan. Heat over low fire, stirring until butter melts and the sauce is hot. Add carrots, and shake the pan until carrots are coated with glaze mixture.

Carrots Hong Kong

4 to 6 Servings

1 pound small, young
   carrots
¼ cup sugar
2 teaspoons cornstarch

1 can (8¾ ounces)
   pineapple spears
1 tablespoon butter
Salt

Wash and carefully scrape carrots. Cut in thin rounds, and cook in boiling salted water for about 20 to 25 minutes. Drain, and set aside.

Mix the sugar and cornstarch together, then stir in pineapple spears, along with the juice from the can. Add butter, and cook over low heat about 4 minutes, until the sauce becomes smooth and begins to thicken. Add the cooked carrots and salt to taste, and continue cooking over low heat until the carrots are warmed through.

Carrots Vichy

4 Servings

1 pound small, young
   carrots
¼ cup water

2 tablespoons butter
1 teaspoon sugar
Salt to taste

Wash and scrape carrots; slice in paper-thin rounds. Place in *heavy* saucepan, together with other ingredients; cover tightly, and cook over low flame. In about 20 minutes the water should be completely evaporated, and the carrots should be cooked and just beginning to glaze.

Celery Cybele

Few American women cook celery, but the adventurous one who cooks for the ulcer dieter should try this recipe. Celery, when *cooked,* is nonacid and has a plus-alkaline factor.

1 bunch young celery	1 cup boiling water
Salt	1 tablespoon butter
1 vegetable bouillon cube	

Wash celery, carefully scrape to remove strings, and cut off leaves. Cut celery lengthwise through heart, making 4 pieces. Cut in half, if necessary, to fit into a shallow casserole that has a cover. Arrange celery in bottom of casserole and sprinkle with salt. Dissolve bouillon cube in boiling water, and add only enough bouillon to cover celery. Dot with butter. Cover, and bake in 375° oven for one hour.

Stewed Cucumbers

2 cucumbers	2 tablespoons butter, melted
½ to ¾ cup clear chicken broth	Salt

Peel and cut cucumbers in small cubes. Put into a saucepan with enough chicken broth to keep the vegetables from burning. Cover, and bring to a boil; then reduce heat to simmer, and cook until tender—about 15 minutes. Serve with melted butter and a dash of salt, if needed.

Scalloped Cucumbers

3 to 4 Servings

Cooked cucumbers are delicious and are perfectly acceptable for an ulcer patient.

3 cucumbers	1½ teaspoons salt
4 to 5 tablespoons butter	¾ cup breadcrumbs
6 tablespoons hot water	

Peel the cucumbers, and slice in thin rounds. Arrange cucumber slices flat in a large shallow baking dish.

Melt 3 tablespoons butter in 6 tablespoons hot water, and pour mixture over cucumbers. Sprinkle with 1½ teaspoons salt. Cover, and bake in 350° preheated oven for 30 minutes.

Remove dish from oven, and sprinkle cucumbers with the breadcrumbs, dotting with the remaining butter. Return dish to oven, uncovered this time, and bake for an additional 25 to 30 minutes, until most of the liquid has been absorbed and the dish is browned on top. Serve immediately.

Eggplant and Chicken-Liver Casserole

6 Servings

2 medium-size eggplants	½ cup grated Parmesan cheese
¼ pound chicken livers	Salt
2 eggs	½ cup breadcrumbs
⅓ cup heavy cream	1 tablespoon butter

Peel eggplants, and cut in small cubes. Cook in boiling salted water for about 10 minutes, or until tender. Drain very well, and set aside.

Broil the chicken livers until just barely done. Remove from broiler, and chop fine.

Put the eggs, cream, cheese, and salt to taste in a blender, and blend for a few seconds until well mixed.

Combine the eggplant cubes, chopped chicken livers, and the blender mixture. Mix well, and spoon into a lightly buttered 1-quart casserole. Top with breadcrumbs, and dot with butter. Bake in 350° oven for 30 minutes.

Scalloped Eggplant de Luxe

4 to 6 Servings

1 eggplant
About ½ cup dry white wine (you may need a bit more)
2 eggs, slightly beaten

1 cup breadcrumbs
5 tablespoons butter, melted
Salt
½ cup grated mild American cheese

Peel eggplant, and cut in small cubes. Place cubes in a saucepan, cover with wine, and cook slowly until tender—about 10 minutes. Remove from heat, and add beaten eggs, breadcrumbs, melted butter, and salt to taste. Mix very well, and spoon into a shallow, buttered baking dish. Top with cheese, and bake in 350° oven for 30 minutes, or until lightly browned.

Endives Parisienne

2 Servings

The use of endives as a cooked vegetable, rather than raw as in a salad, is very common in France and Belgium. Endives have a vaguely bitter taste, which may not appeal to the younger family members; but try this recipe on the man-in-your-life for vegetable variety.

4 endives	4 tablespoons butter
1 can clear chicken broth	Salt

Wash endives, remove outer leaves, and trim bottoms. If the endives are very large, slice in two lengthwise. Put in a skillet, and pour in enough chicken broth so it is about ½-inch deep. Cover, and bring to a boil. Turn heat down, and simmer about 20 minutes.

Drain endives, and add 4 tablespoons butter (you may need more if endives are large). Cover, and simmer over very low heat another 10 minutes. Salt sparingly before serving.

Braised Endives

4 Servings

8 endives	1 tablespoon lemon juice
3 tablespoons butter	Salt

Wash the endives, and trim off any discolored tips. Boil in salted water for 10 minutes.

While endives are boiling, melt the butter in the top of a small double boiler, and add lemon juice.

Arrange the parboiled endives in a single layer in a shallow baking dish. Pour the butter and lemon sauce over them, and turn the endives once with tongs so they are coated with the sauce. Sprinkle lightly with salt, and bake in 325° oven for 1 hour, turning once.

Minorcan Hearts of Palm

4 Servings

1 can (14 ounces) hearts of palm	1 cup milk
3 tablespoons butter	Salt
2 tablespoons flour	3 tablespoons breadcrumbs

Set oven at 350°.

Drain hearts of palm, and place in a shallow baking dish.

Melt 2 tablespoons butter in the top of a double boiler. When melted, stir in flour and mix well. Add milk and salt to taste, and stir constantly until sauce is smooth and begins to thicken.

Pour sauce over hearts of palm, sprinkle breadcrumbs on top, and dot with remaining 1 tablespoon butter. Bake in preheated oven for 20 minutes or until light brown and bubbly. Serve immediately.

Pea Purée

4 Servings

2 packages frozen tiny peas   ½ cup heavy cream
1 tablespoon butter   Salt

Cook peas in a saucepan according to directions on package. When done, drain, and put in blender to purée. When puréed, return to saucepan, and heat over very low heat until the purée is quite dry. Add butter, heavy cream, and salt to taste. Stir constantly until butter is melted and cream is thoroughly heated.

Casserole of Spinach

6 Servings

2 packages frozen chopped   4 tablespoons butter
  spinach   Salt
1 package (8 ounces) cream   1 cup breadcrumbs
  cheese

Cook spinach according to directions on package, and drain very well.

Soften cream cheese, and mix spinach with the cheese, 2 tablespoons butter, and salt to taste. Stir well to combine thoroughly. Spoon into a 1½-quart casserole.

Melt the remaining 2 tablespoons butter in the top of a double boiler. When melted, toss with breadcrumbs, and sprinkle mixture over the spinach. Bake in 350° oven for 20 minutes, or until mixture bubbles and is lightly browned.

High Spinach Soufflé

4 to 6 Servings

2 packages frozen chopped spinach	1 cup milk
	Salt
2 tablespoons butter	1 egg yolk
2 tablespoons flour	3 egg whites

Preheat oven to 375°.

Cook spinach according to directions on package. Drain very well.

Meanwhile, melt butter in the top of a double boiler. When melted, stir in flour and blend well. Stir in milk and salt to taste. Cook for about 5 minutes, stirring constantly. When sauce starts to thicken, mix in the spinach and egg yolk. Stir well. Cool 15 minutes.

Beat egg whites until they are stiff; fold into cooled spinach mixture. Carefully turn into a 1½-quart soufflé dish, and bake in 375° oven for 30 minutes.

As with all soufflés, *serve immediately* after removing from oven.

Honey-Baked Acorn Squash

4 Servings

2 medium-size acorn squash Salt
2 tablespoons butter, melted ¼ cup honey

Halve each squash lengthwise, and scoop out seeds. Brush inside surfaces with 1 tablespoon melted butter, and sprinkle with salt. Put squash in shallow pan, with the cut sides down. Bake in 375° oven for 30 minutes, then turn.

Combine remaining 1 tablespoon melted butter with honey. Brush over hollows in the squash. Continue baking for another 30 minutes, or until squash is tender.

Pilgrim Squash

4 Servings

2 acorn squash ⅓ cup cranberry jelly
⅓ cup butter, melted

Cut squash in half lengthwise, and remove seeds. Place in a baking pan, with cut sides down. Bake in 350° oven for 45 minutes.

Meanwhile, combine the butter and jelly, blending well. When 45 minutes' baking time is up, turn squash, and spoon the butter and jelly mixture into the centers. Bake an additional 15 minutes, or until tender.

Squash Medley

4 Servings

2 small summer squash
2 small zucchini
4 tablespoons butter, melted

Salt
2 tablespoons orange juice

Wash summer squash and zucchini, peel, and slice in thin rounds. Arrange in a lightly buttered baking dish.

Pour melted butter over vegetables, and mix lightly. Sprinkle with salt to taste. Bake in 350° oven for 25 minutes, or until vegetables are tender.

Sprinkle with orange juice, and stir gently until blended. Return to oven for 5 minutes.

Zucchini Provencal

4 Servings

4 zucchini
3 small tomatoes, peeled
Salt

2 tablespoons pure olive oil
3 tablespoons grated
   Parmesan cheese

Wash and *lightly* scrape the zucchini, then cut in two lengthwise. Trim zucchini at both ends, but keep the shells intact. With a paring knife, criss-cross the pulp within the shells, then put the zucchini into boiling water, and cook for 3 minutes.

Drain zucchini, and carefully remove the pulp. Set the

shells in a buttered baking dish.

Chop the zucchini pulp and the peeled tomatoes. Lightly salt vegetables. Combine, and simmer this mixture in the top of a double boiler, with the olive oil, for 15 minutes. Fill zucchini shells with pulp and tomato mixtures. Sprinkle with grated Parmesan cheese, and bake in 350° oven for 15 minutes, or until lightly browned.

Zucchini-Tomato Bake

4 Servings

4 small zucchini
3 small tomatoes
Salt

2 tablespoons water
1 cup breadcrumbs
2 tablespoons butter

Wash, pare, and slice zucchini in thin rounds. Wash, peel, and slice tomatoes. Lightly salt vegetables.

In a buttered baking dish put one layer of sliced zucchini, then one layer of sliced tomatoes. Continue until all vegetables are used. Add 2 tablespoons water. Top with breadcrumbs and butter. Bake in 375° oven for 45 minutes.

String Beans Mimosa

4 Servings

2 packages frozen string
   beans, French style
2 hard-cooked eggs

2 tablespoons butter, melted
Salt

Cook beans according to directions on package. Keep warm.

Halve hard-cooked eggs, and separate yolks from whites. Press yolks through a sieve, then press whites through a sieve.

Put cooked beans in serving bowl, and sprinkle with egg yolks, then egg whites. Drizzle melted butter over all. Add salt to taste, and serve.

Tomato Stuffed with Broccoli

4 Servings

This recipe is *only* for those who are well on the way to recovery. Some patients find broccoli hard to digest, and all should avoid eating the tomato skins.

4 medium-size tomatoes
1 package frozen chopped
    broccoli
½ cup milk
1½ tablespoons flour

1½ tablespoons butter
Salt
¼ cup breadcrumbs
2 tablespoons grated
    Parmesan cheese

Cut the tops off the tomatoes, and scoop out the insides. Turn tomatoes upside down to drain.

Cook chopped broccoli according to directions on package. Drain. Put broccoli in blender with milk, flour, butter, and salt to taste. Blend until broccoli is puréed and well mixed with other ingredients.

Fill tomatoes with puréed broccoli, top with breadcrumbs and Parmesan cheese. Arrange tomatoes in a lightly buttered baking dish, and bake in 350° oven for 30 minutes, or until golden brown on top. Do not overcook, as tomatoes tend to fall apart when cooked too long.

Fountain-of-Youth Casserole

4 Servings

2 large firm tomatoes, peeled
1 cup potatoes, peeled and
   thinly sliced
1 cup carrots, scraped and
   thinly sliced

1 cup summer squash,
   scraped and thinly sliced
Salt
1 tablespoon water
2 tablespoons butter

Wash all vegetables, and prepare according to directions given above. Slice tomatoes into slices about ½-inch thick.

Lightly butter a casserole—one that has a tight cover. Place vegetables in layers, with tomatoes on the bottom. Sprinkle each layer with a pinch of salt. Sprinkle 1 tablespoon water over all, and dot with butter. Cover, and bake in 375° oven for 1 hour.

Pasta and Rice

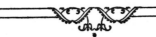

Noodles, macaroni, and spaghetti are fine foods for the ulcer patient, as long as they are not served with sauces that contain onions, garlic, parsley, clams, black or red pepper, green pepper, or unpeeled tomatoes. After all, there is no law—not even in Italy—that requires every pasta dish to be topped with a spicy tomato-sauce mixture.

Rice also is a starch that ulcer patients have no trouble digesting—provided it is not served with traditionally made chicken or beef gravy. (Rice contains acid-forming elements, but in less quantity than beef or eggs.) You might try our Yorkshire Rice recipe, page 141, with roast beef. It's a good substitute for Yorkshire Pudding, which the ulcer patient must avoid. In all our rice recipes, unless otherwise specified, either natural rice or packaged, precooked rice may be used.

In any discussion of foods containing starch, the matter of calories nearly always comes to mind. Actually, very few ulcer patients need to be calorie conscious. High-strung, animated individuals (the typical ulcer patient) burn off calories very quickly, and they need some starch, which the body converts into glucose, for energy.

The pasta recipes in this chapter can be used as a main dish for a light weekend luncheon, or instead of potatoes at dinner. A practical rule when menu planning is to serve elaborate pasta and rice recipes with simple meat and vegetable dishes.

Spring Noodle Ring

6 Servings

1 cup medium-size, uncooked
   noodles
1½ cups hot milk
1 cup breadcrumbs
¼ cup butter, melted

Salt
6 egg yolks, beaten
1½ cups grated Parmesan
   cheese

Break noodles into small pieces before cooking in boiling salted water, following directions on box. Drain, and rinse with a dash of cold water. Combine noodles with milk, breadcrumbs, butter, and salt to taste. Add beaten egg yolks and cheese. Mix thoroughly.

Spoon into a buttered 8-inch ring mold, and place mold in a pan of hot water. Bake in 350° oven until firm and golden on top—45 minutes to an hour. This dish should be firm but fluffy.

Unmold and serve. Fill center with cooked asparagus tips, if desired.

Venetian Macaroni

6 Servings

2 cups uncooked elbow
   macaroni
6 firm, medium-size
   tomatoes
2 tablespoons butter
2 tablespoons flour

1 cup milk
½ cup grated Parmesan
   cheese
½ cup breadcrumbs
Salt

Cook macaroni according to directions on box. Drain, rinse, and set aside.

Cut tops off the tomatoes, scoop out pulp, and drain by turning upside down. (Pulp can be saved for soup.)

Melt butter in the top of a double boiler. Blend in flour; add milk, stirring constantly, until sauce is smooth and begins to thicken. Add cheese, and stir. Remove from heat, and mix with macaroni. Add salt to taste.

Fill the tomatoes with the mixture and top with breadcrumbs. Dot with butter. Bake in 350° oven for 45 minutes.

Remember, the ulcer patient must not eat skin of tomato.

Macaroni Rarebit

6 Servings

2 cups uncooked elbow
  macaroni
2 tablespoons butter
3 cups grated mild
  American cheese

3 egg yolks
¾ cup milk
Salt
4 to 6 slices white bread,
  toasted

Cook macaroni according to directions on box. Drain, and rinse with a dash of cold water. Set aside.

Melt butter in the top of a large double boiler; add cheese, and stir until cheese is melted. Beat egg yolks with the milk, and add to cheese mixture, stirring until smooth. Add salt to taste. Stir in cooked macaroni, and mix well. Heat for 10 minutes. Serve over slices of toast.

Spaghetti au Gratin

4 Servings

1 box (8 ounces) spaghetti
1 cup grated Parmesan
  cheese

1 cup cream
2 tablespoons butter

Cook spaghetti in salted water, following directions on box. Place a layer of spaghetti in a lightly buttered 1-quart baking dish, then a layer of cheese, then another layer of spaghetti, and so on, until spaghetti and cheese are used up. Pour on cream, and dot with butter. Bake in 350° oven for 35 minutes, or until golden brown.

Spaghetti la Scala

4 Servings

1 box (8 ounces) thin
  spaghetti
1 can cream of vegetable
  soup or cream of celery
  soup
½ cup milk

½ cup our mayonnaise
  (page 197)
Salt
2 hard-cooked eggs, peeled
  and sliced
2 tablespoons grated mild
  American cheese

Cook spaghetti according to directions on box. Drain, and rinse with a dash of cold water. Place in a lightly buttered 1-quart baking dish.

Combine the soup, milk, and mayonnaise in a saucepan; heat slowly until the mixture is smooth and hot. Add salt to taste. Stir half the sauce into the spaghetti.

Place hard-cooked egg slices over spaghetti, and pour remaining sauce over all. Top with grated cheese. Bake in 350° oven for 30 minutes, or until light brown and bubbly.

Spaghetti Soufflé

6 Servings

1 box (8 ounces) spaghetti
4 tablespoons butter
4 tablespoons flour

2 cups milk
Salt
5 eggs, separated

Break spaghetti into small pieces. Cook according to directions on box, following instructions for firm spaghetti. Drain, rinse with a dash of cold water, and set aside.

Melt butter in the top of a double boiler. Blend in flour, then add milk, stirring constantly until mixture is smooth and begins to thicken. Add salt to taste.

Beat egg yolks until light, and slowly add to white sauce, stirring all the while. Blend this mixture into cooked spaghetti. Set aside to cool slightly.

Beat egg whites until stiff but not dry. When spaghetti has cooled (about 15 minutes), fold in stiff egg whites. Spoon mixture into a lightly buttered 1-quart soufflé dish, and bake in 375° oven for 30 minutes, or until puffy and lightly browned on top. Serve at once.

Baked Ravioli

4 Servings

24 frozen meat-filled ravioli,
  1 package
3 tablespoons butter
3 tablespoons flour

2 cups milk
Salt
4 teaspoons grated
  Parmesan cheese

Cook frozen ravioli according to directions on package, but shorten cooking time by 5 minutes. Drain, and set aside.

Melt butter in the top of a double boiler. When melted, stir in flour, and blend very well. Add milk, and stir constantly until mixture is smooth and begins to thicken. Add salt to taste.

Lightly butter 4 ramekins, and put 6 ravioli in the bottom of each. Pour sauce mixture over ravioli, then top each dish with 1 teaspoon grated cheese. Bake in 350° oven for 30 minutes, or until lightly browned.

Yorkshire Rice

6 Servings

2 cups cooked rice
1 egg
2 cups milk
Salt

1 cup grated mild American
  cheese
½ cup breadcrumbs

Cook rice according to directions on box.

Put egg, milk, cooked rice, and a pinch of salt in a blender, and blend for 5 to 10 seconds until very well mixed. Add cheese and breadcrumbs, and blend again to combine all ingredients. *Mixture will be very thin.*

Pour into a lightly buttered 1-quart soufflé dish, and bake in 325° oven for 45 minutes, or until lightly browned.

Arroz Redondo

---

6 Servings

3 cups cooked rice
¼ pound mild American
   cheese, grated

1 cup commercial sour
   cream
Salt

Cook rice according to directions on box.

Toss the cooked rice and cheese together in a large bowl. Fold in the sour cream. Add salt to taste. Spoon mixture into a 4-cup ring mold, packing it down lightly. Bake in 350° oven for 30 minutes.

After removing from oven, cool in the mold for 5 minutes. Unmold by running a knife around the edge and center of the ring. Cover with a serving plate, turn upside down, and lift off the mold.

Riz Rose

---

6 Servings

3 cups cooked rice
4 eggs, hard-cooked
1 can (3¼ ounces) sardines
   (not tomato packed)
1 tablespoon our
   mayonnaise (page 197)

Salt
2 tablespoons butter
1 tablespoon flour
1 can tomato soup
½ cup water

Cook rice according to directions on box.

Split hard-cooked eggs lengthwise, scoop out yolks and add to sardines. Mash together, and blend in mayonnaise and salt to taste. Spoon this stuffing into the egg-white halves.

Melt butter in the top of a double boiler, add flour, and blend. Add tomato soup (undiluted) and water, stirring until mixture thickens.

Spoon rice into a buttered 1-quart baking dish, and pour about ¾ of the tomato sauce on top. (Keep remaining sauce warm.) Arrange the stuffed eggs on the rice, and bake in 350° oven for 30 minutes. When removing from oven, pour rest of tomato sauce, in ribbon fashion, over the dish for garnish.

Rice and Tuna Pie

6 Servings

2 cups cooked rice
2 tablespoons butter
1 egg, slightly beaten
1 can (7 ounces) tuna in
    water pack, drained

3 eggs, beaten
1 cup milk
1 cup shredded Swiss cheese
Salt

Cook rice according to directions on box.

Combine the rice, butter, and egg. Press into bottom and sides of a lightly buttered 10-inch pie pan. Sprinkle drained tuna evenly over this rice shell.

Combine remaining ingredients, and pour over tuna. Bake in 350° oven for 50 to 55 minutes, until a knife inserted just off-center comes out clean.

Rice au Gratin in a Minute

2 Servings

1⅓ cups packaged pre-
    cooked rice

¾ cup grated mild
    American cheese
2 tablespoons butter

Cook rice according to directions on box. When done, place rice in 1½-quart casserole, top with grated cheese, and dot with butter. Bake in 350° oven, about 15 minutes, or until cheese melts and is lightly browned.

Riz-Fromage Casserole

6 Servings

1 cup rice (do *not* use
    packaged precooked rice)
1 envelope *dry* chicken-rice
    soup mix
2½ cups water

⅔ cup evaporated milk
1 can cream of chicken soup
1 cup American cheese,
    cubed

Combine rice, dry soup mix, and water in a saucepan. Bring to boil. Cover tightly, and simmer, according to directions on rice box. (Remember, do *not* use packaged precooked rice.)

When rice is done, add milk, cream of chicken soup (undiluted), and cheese. Mix well. Spoon into a lightly buttered casserole. Bake in 350° oven for 30 minutes, or until light brown on top.

Cajun Rice

6 Servings

1½ cups rice (do *not* use
    packaged precooked rice)
1½ cups cut-up tomatoes,
    peeled

1 can clear chicken broth
2 tablespoons butter
Salt

Put rice, cut-up tomatoes, chicken broth, and butter into a saucepan that has a lid. Bring to boil, cover, and cook according to timing directions on rice box—or until liquid is absorbed. Add a dash of salt if necessary, and fluff before serving.

Eggs and Cheese

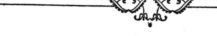

Eggs are great for the ulcer patient, but never fried, please. You can serve eggs boiled, poached, scrambled in the top of a double boiler, or hard-cooked.

Many cookbooks fail to give instructions on how to hard-cook an egg, so we will: Put the eggs in a saucepan with enough cold water to completely cover them, and add a few drops of vinegar. This will help to prevent the eggshells from cracking. Bring the water to a rapid boil, reduce the heat until the water is simmering. Cook for 10 or 12 minutes—eggs really do not need to be cooked longer than that. Drain, plunge into cold water, and when cool enough to handle, peel.

Generally, we prefer to avoid omelets since the conventional method of preparation involves pan-frying. However, many later-stage patients are able to digest omelets without any after-effects, so we have included one recipe in this popular and palatable category.

Our cheese recipes are versatile, some of them hearty enough to substitute for meat dishes. All were developed with mild cheese, which is advisable. Processed mild American cheddar is not an elegant cheese, but it melts easily, has a creamy texture, keeps very well, and doesn't tax the digestive system.

Baked Omelet

4 Servings

3 tablespoons dry
   breadcrumbs
1 cup milk

5 eggs, separated
Salt

Soak the breadcrumbs in the milk for 1 hour. Lightly beat egg yolks. Stir the breadcrumbs into the yolks, and season with salt to taste. Beat egg whites until stiff but not dry, and fold into mixture.

Butter a deep (2½ to 3-inch) baking dish, and pour the mixture into it. Place on the lower rack of a 375° oven, and bake for 30 minutes until puffy and light brown. Serve at once.

Eggs Andalusia

2 to 4 Servings

4 eggs, poached
1 tablespoon sherry
1 tablespoon butter
3 tablespoons clear chicken
   broth

4 tablespoons heavy cream
4 tablespoons grated
   Parmesan cheese

Poach eggs as you usually do.

Meanwhile, simmer sherry, butter, and chicken broth for 5 minutes, then pour into a 9-inch glass pie pan.

With a large perforated spoon, transfer poached eggs to pie pan. Spoon 1 tablespoon heavy cream over each egg, and top with Parmesan cheese. Put under broiler until golden. Serve immediately.

Eggs Primavera

4 Servings

2 packages frozen chopped
spinach
4 eggs, poached

1 can chicken noodle soup

Cook spinach according to directions on package, and drain very well. Warm a 1½-quart baking dish, and then line with spinach. With a large spoon, make 4 depressions in the spinach.

Poach eggs as you usually do. Using a perforated spoon, place 1 poached egg in each depression.

Put chicken noodle soup (undiluted) in a blender and whirl until smooth—about 20 seconds. Pour soup over eggs and spinach, and put under broiler until bubbly and lightly browned. Serve immediately.

Daffodil Eggs

6 Servings

6 eggs, hard-cooked
1 cup butter, melted
Salt

2 cups Sauce Verte (page
198)
6 pieces of bread

Cut hard-cooked eggs in half, and separate whites from yolks. Chop the whites very well, and press through a fine sieve. Melt butter in the top of a double boiler, and season with a little salt. Mix egg whites with the butter and keep hot.

Sieve the yolks so they are practically a yellow powder, and set aside.

Make Sauce Verte according to instructions on page 198. Toast 6 pieces of bread, and butter lightly. Cover the bread (don't drown) with the spinach sauce. Arrange toast on a platter, and cover each piece with the egg-white mixture. Finally, put a spoonful of the sieved egg yolks in the center of each piece of toast.

Nesting Eggs

4 Servings

This turn-of-the-century recipe is as good today as it was then; a treat for brunch or lunch.

4 tablespoons butter	1 tablespoon flour
6 eggs, hard-cooked	1 teaspoon salt
6 to 8 stalks celery	1 can (7 ounces) tuna in
2 cups milk	water pack

Melt butter in the top of a double boiler, and set aside.

Separate the hard-cooked egg whites from the yolks. Cut whites into long thin strips; set yolks aside. Place egg-white strips around the edges of a large, flat buttered baking dish. Set the oven at 200° or "warm," and put the dish inside to heat.

Shred celery, put in a small saucepan with 1 cup of the milk, and bring to a boil. Reduce heat, add ½ teaspoon salt, and simmer for about 25 minutes, until the celery is stewed tender and most of the liquid has been absorbed.

Remove dish from oven, and spoon celery inside the ring of egg whites. Pour 2 tablespoons melted butter over both ingredients. Place dish in warm oven.

Return the double boiler (with the remaining melted butter) to heat. Add 1 tablespoon flour and remaining ½ teaspoon salt, stirring until blended; then slowly add remaining cup of milk, stirring all the while. Let cook for 5 minutes until well blended and thickened. Remove from heat.

Drain the tuna. Press egg yolks through a sieve, then mix well with the fish, adding 2 tablespoons of the sauce. Form fish mixture into small egg-shaped balls.

Remove dish from oven, and place these balls neatly inside the "nest" of egg whites. Pour the rest of the sauce over all. Turn oven up to 350°, and reheat dish for 10 minutes, until well heated all the way through. Serve at once.

Frothy Asparagus Eggs

2 Servings if for lunch
4 Servings if side dish

1 can (8 ounces) asparagus spears and tips	Salt
4 eggs	1 cup milk
2 tablespoons butter	1 can (16½ ounces) green asparagus tips
1 tablespoon flour	

Set oven at 350°.

Drain can of asparagus tips. Beat eggs well and set aside.

In the top of a double boiler, melt buter; add flour and salt, stirring all the while. Add milk gradually and continue stirring. Let sauce cook for 5 minutes until well blended and thickened. Remove from heat. Pour sauce slowly into the beaten eggs, stirring constantly; add the drained asparagus spears and tips.

Drain the can of asparagus tips. Butter a medium-size baking dish and line with the green tips. Pour in the asparagus-and-sauce mixture. Place the dish in a pan of water and bake in preheated 350° oven for about 45 minutes. Serve immediately.

South-of-the-Border Eggs

4 Servings

1 package dried beef
1 cup canned peeled
   tomatoes, drained and cut
   into small pieces

¼ cup grated Parmesan
   cheese
Few drops of lemon juice
2 tablespoons butter
3 eggs, well-beaten

Cut the dried beef into fine strips with scissors. Combine with tomatoes, cheese, and lemon juice.

Melt butter in the top of a double boiler. Add everything except the eggs, and cook for 5 minutes. Then pour in the well-beaten eggs and cook, stirring constantly, until eggs have a creamy consistency, like moist scrambled eggs.

Sunny Tomato Eggs

2 Servings

2 *large* tomatoes	Salt
2 teaspoons butter, melted	2 eggs

Peel tomatoes. (If you prefer, leave the skin on, but be sure the patient doesn't eat it.) Cut tops off tomatoes. In the center of each, make a hollow large enough to hold an egg. This means discarding quite a bit of the center tomato pulp, almost to the fleshy walls, but it is necessary; otherwise the egg will slop over, and you lose most of the white.

Put a teaspoon of melted butter in the hollow of each tomato, and add a dash of salt. Break one egg (break them separately in a cup first, to be sure they are fresh) into each hollow. Place the tomatoes on a buttered cookie sheet or in a flat ovenproof dish, and bake in 350° oven for 30 minutes, until eggs are firm and tomatoes cooked.

American Soufflé

2 Servings

1 tablespoon butter	½ cup grated mild
2 tablespoons flour	American cheese
½ cup milk	Salt
	2 eggs, separated

Set oven at 350°.

Melt butter in the top of a double boiler. Stir in flour and blend well. Add milk, stirring constantly, until the mixture is smooth. Add grated cheese. Continue cooking until cheese has melted. Add salt to taste. Remove from heat, and cool for about 10 minutes.

While the cheese mixture is cooling, beat egg yolks with a whisk or a fork, until they are light and frothy. Beat egg whites with an electric beater, until they are stiff and stand in firm peaks.

Add well-beaten egg yolks to the cheese mixture, and blend well. Then carefully fold in the stiff egg whites. Pour into a 2-cup soufflé dish. Place the soufflé dish in a pan of hot water and bake in 350° oven for 1 hour. Serve at once.

Do not open oven door to look at the soufflé during cooking time. If air gets into the oven, no soufflé can rise and crown properly.

Sunday-Night Soufflé

4 Servings

1 can cream of celery soup   6 eggs, separated
1 cup grated mild American
  cheese

Set oven at 350°.

Combine soup (undiluted) with grated cheese, and heat slowly until cheese melts. Remove from heat, and set aside to cool slightly.

Meanwhile, beat egg yolks until thick and lemon-colored. Beat egg whites with an electric beater until stiff but not dry.

Add yolks to soup-and-cheese mixture. Carefully fold in egg whites. Pour into a 2-quart soufflé dish, and bake in 350° oven for 50 minutes. Serve immediately.

Remember, soufflés are shy and will not puff up properly if the oven door is opened during baking time.

Pots of Gold

4 Servings

2 packages (3 ounces
    each) cream cheese
¾ cup milk

4 eggs
Salt

Heat the cream cheese in the top of a double boiler until it is soft.

Put milk, eggs, and salt to taste in a blender and blend for a few seconds. Add the soft cream cheese, and blend until all ingredients are well mixed. Pour into 4 custard cups, and bake in a pan of hot water in 375° oven for 25 minutes.

Strata

6 Servings

12 slices day-old bread
6 slices processed American
    cheese, sliced

4 eggs
2½ cups milk
Salt

Trim the crusts from the bread. Arrange 6 slices in the bottom of a 12 x 7 x 2-inch flat baking dish. Cover each piece of bread with a slice of cheese, then top with remaining pieces of bread.

Beat eggs; add milk and salt to taste. Pour over bread and cheese. Let stand 1 hour.

Bake in 325° oven for 1 hour. Serve immediately.

Lunar Custard

2 egg yolks
2 cups grated mild
American cheese

½ cup milk
Dash of salt

Set oven at 300°.

Beat egg yolks until light, then add remaining ingredients, and stir. Pour mixture into buttered individual baking dishes. Place in pan of hot water, and bake in preheated oven about 25 minutes, or until the eggs are set.

Spaghetti and Cheese Custard

1 box (8 ounces) thin
spaghetti
3 eggs
⅓ cup butter
1½ cups milk

Salt
½ pound mild American
cheese, cut into small
pieces
½ cup breadcrumbs

Break spaghetti in half, or into smaller pieces, and cook according to directions on package. Drain, and put in a large mixing bowl.

Put the eggs, butter, milk, salt to taste, and cheese in a blender, and blend for about 30 seconds. Pour sauce over spaghetti, and mix lightly but well.

Place mixture in a lightly buttered flat 9 x 12-inch baking dish. Top with breadcrumbs. Set baking dish in a pan of hot water, and bake in 350° oven for 1 hour, or until the custard has set.

Salads

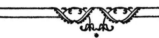

Ulcer patients do not need to forgo salads, nor should they. But they do need to eat a "different" type of salad. In this chapter we are presenting nineteen recipes, utilizing plenty of cooked fruits and vegetables in order to provide the necessary A, B, and C vitamins. Vitamin C is especially important for ulcer graduates, since colds seem to trigger ulcer symptoms in many former patients.

Try our salad recipes, and before long your ulcer dieter won't be unhappy about giving up lettuce, cucumbers, tomatoes, radishes—any of the raw vegetables used in salads. Other members of the family should add lettuce and/or fresh fruit to their portions. The normal digestive system needs the roughage that salad greens supply.

A brief comment about salad dressing for molded salads: Ulcer patients should not be served commercial mayonnaise, which contains mustard, vinegar, and preservatives. We recommend our special Mandalay House mayonnaise recipe on page 197. Our mayonnaise is quick to make (a matter of seconds) and easy to digest. This dressing is equally good when made with high-grade pure olive oil or with poly-unsaturated oil.

If you have had trouble unmolding salads this could be due to the fact that you are not following directions accurately. You may be using too much or too little gelatin, or not dissolving it properly. When unmolding, remember to quickly dip your mold into a pan of hot water, clap a plate or platter on top of the mold, and invert. And as one well-known cook and television personality said: It also helps to pray!

Asparagus in Celery Jelly

6 Servings

2 cups celery, finely diced
2 young carrots, finely diced
2 cups water
Salt
2 tablespoons unflavored
    gelatin
¼ cup cold water

1 can (10½ ounces)
    asparagus tips
Liquid from the can of
    asparagus
Our mayonnaise for garnish
    (page 197)

Wash and scrape the celery and carrots; dice. Cook in 2 cups water, salted to taste, for 15 minutes. Drain, but *reserve* 1 cup of the cooking liquid. Chill celery and carrots.

Soften the gelatin in ¼ cup cold water. Open can of asparagus tips, drain, but *reserve* liquid from can. Add enough water to the asparagus liquid to make 1 cup. Add this to the 1 cup of celery-carrot stock. Heat just to boiling, add softened gelatin, and stir.

Pour a thin layer of gelatin mixture into a long mold, approximately 8 x 4 x 2 inches, and chill until sticky-firm. Keep remaining gelatin mixture at room temperature.

When gelatin in mold is slightly firm, add a layer of asparagus tips, cooked celery, and carrots. Pour on the rest of the gelatin mixture, and chill for several hours. To serve, unmold and garnish with our mayonnaise.

Asparagus Jockey Club

4 Servings

16 cold cooked asparagus
spears
2 hard-cooked eggs, finely
chopped

Salt
4 teaspoons our mayonnaise
(page 197)

Arrange 4 spears of asparagus on each salad plate. Sprinkle with finely chopped hard-cooked egg and salt to taste. Top each with 1 teaspoon our mayonnaise.

Russian Mold

4 to 6 Servings

1 can (8¼ ounces) diced
beets
1 package lime gelatin
1 cup boiling water
½ cup beet juice from can
½ cup cold water

3 tablespoons lemon juice
½ teaspoon salt
4 to 6 tablespoons
commercial sour cream
for topping

Drain can of beets, saving juice.

Dissolve gelatin in 1 cup boiling water, add ½ cup beet juice, ½ cup cold water, lemon juice, and salt. Pour into 4-cup mold and chill until gelatin is just starting to set. (This can take up to 2 hours.)

When gelatin is beginning to firm, add drained beets and mix into gelatin mixture. Return to refrigerator, and chill until firm.

Unmold, and serve with sour-cream topping.

Cheese and Pineapple Ring

8 Servings

3 cups cottage cheese
1 cup crushed pineapple,
   drained
5 tablespoons our
   mayonnaise (page 197)

2 tablespoons lemon juice
1 teaspoon salt
1½ tablespoons unflavored
   gelatin
1 cup pineapple juice

Mix cottage cheese, pineapple, and mayonnaise. Add lemon juice and salt. Mix lightly.

Soften gelatin in pineapple juice, and dissolve in the top of a double boiler. Stir dissolved gelatin and pineapple juice into cheese mixture. Turn into medium-size mold, and chill until firm.

Chicken Salad Oahu

4 Servings

2 cups cooked chicken,
   cut into small cubes
1 can (8¾ ounces) pineapple
   spears, drained

4 tablespoons our
   mayonnaise (page 197)
Lemon juice
Salt

Combine chicken cubes, pineapple spears, and mayonnaise. When mixing, add a dash of lemon juice and salt to taste. Chill well before serving.

Salade Imperatrice

4 Servings

2 cups cold cooked rice
½ cup our mayonnaise (page 197)
1 tablespoon sugar
1 cup cooked chicken, diced

1 tablespoon lemon juice
1 tablespoon cream
1 tablespoon pineapple juice or orange juice
Salt

Put all the ingredients into a large bowl and mix well. Pack very tightly into a 1-quart soufflé dish, and chill for 3 hours.

To serve, put serving platter over the top of the soufflé dish, and quickly turn over. If salad has been packed tightly and chilled long enough, it will unmold easily.

Turkey-Cranberry Mold

4 to 6 Servings

1 tablespoon unflavored gelatin
¼ cup cold water
⅔ cup cranberry jelly

1½ cups boiling water
2 cups cold cooked turkey, diced

Soak the gelatin in cold water for 5 minutes. Melt the cranberry jelly in the top of a double boiler, stirring constantly; then add the boiling water. Stir in gelatin.

Chill mixture until it starts to thicken; then add the diced turkey, and turn mixture into a mold that has been rinsed in cold water. Chill several hours until firm.

Picnic Egg Aspic

4 to 6 Servings

1 envelope unflavored
gelatin
2 cups clear chicken broth
4 eggs, hard-cooked

3 carrots, cooked
Our mayonnaise for garnish
(page 197)

Soften gelatin in ½ cup cold broth for 5 minutes. Put remaining 1½ cups broth in the top of a double boiler, add softened gelatin, and dissolve over heat.

Pour *half* of this mixture into a long pan or glass baking dish, about 10 x 6 x 2 inches, and chill until firm. Keep remaining half of gelatin mixture at room temperature.

Cut eggs in half, lengthwise. Put eggs, cut side down, on the firm gelatin mixture. Slice cooked carrots into thin rounds, and arrange around eggs. Spoon remaining unchilled gelatin mixture over eggs and carrots. Chill until firm.

Cut into squares, and serve on individual salad plates. Garnish with our mayonnaise.

Jellied Egg and Tongue

4 Servings

¼ pound cooked tongue
4 eggs, hard-cooked
Salt

1 package lemon gelatin
3 tablespoons our
mayonnaise (page 197)

Chop, separately, the cooked tongue and hard-cooked eggs. Salt lightly, and set aside.

Prepare lemon gelatin, following directions on package. Cool until just slightly firm, add chopped tongue, chopped eggs, and mayonnaise. Mix well, turn into a medium-size mold that has been rinsed in cold water, and chill until firm.

Sicilian Egg Salad

4 to 6 Servings

1 cup cooked spinach
2 eggs, hard-cooked
1 package (3 ounces) cream
   cheese
Salt

2 tablespoons olive oil
2 tablespoons lemon juice
Our mayonnaise for garnish
   (page 197)

Chop, separately, the spinach and hard-cooked eggs. When both are chopped to a fine consistency, mix together. Soften cream cheese by working with a large wooden spoon, then add to egg and spinach mixture. Add salt to taste.

Blend oil and lemon juice, add to spinach mixture, and combine very well. Chill until slightly firm. Form into balls, and serve on a bed of lettuce. The patient should not eat the lettuce, of course, but it enhances the appearance of the salad. Garnish with our mayonnaise, if desired.

Stockholm Fish Salad

6 Servings

2 egg *yolks,* hard-cooked
Salt
1 egg *yolk,* uncooked
¼ cup milk
2 tablespoons lemon juice
½ cup heavy cream

2 cups flaked cooked fish
   (leftovers, or drained tuna
   in water pack)
½ cup cooked French-style
   string beans, drained and
   finely chopped
½ cup cooked carrots,
   drained and finely diced

Press hard-cooked egg yolks through a fine sieve, and season with salt to taste. Mix with uncooked egg yolk, milk, and lemon juice. Whip heavy cream until stiff, and add to egg mixture. Gently fold in fish and vegetables. Chill well before serving.

Macaroni Luncheon Salad

4 to 6 Servings

1 box (6 ounces) elbow macaroni

½ cup commercial sour cream

½ cup our mayonnaise (page 197)

1 can (7 ounces) tuna in water pack

1 can (10½ ounces) green beans

¼ cup grated mild American cheese

Salt

Cook the macaroni according to directions on box. Drain, and cool slightly. Stir in sour cream and mayonnaise.

Drain tuna and green beans, then gently mix into macaroni. Add grated cheese and salt to taste. Chill.

Macaroni-Salmon Salad

4 to 6 Servings

2 cups shell macaroni
2 cups salmon
  (about two 7¾-ounce cans
  in water pack)

2 tablespoons lemon juice
1 cup our mayonnaise
  (page 197)
2 hard-cooked eggs, sliced

Cook the macaroni according to directions on box. Drain, and let cool. Meanwhile, drain the salmon and separate into flakes, being sure all bones and skin are removed. When macaroni is cold, mix it with the lemon juice, salmon, and mayonnaise. Form the mixture into a mound on a pretty platter, and garnish with sliced hard-cooked eggs.

Jellied Mandarin Orange and Lime Salad

6 Servings

1 package lime gelatin
1 cup boiling water
1 can (11 ounces) mandarin-
  orange segments

Juice from mandarin-
  orange can
1 avocado, sliced

Dissolve gelatin in 1 cup boiling water.

Drain mandarin-orange segments, *reserving* the juice from the can. Add enough water to the juice to make 1 cup, and add to dissolved gelatin. Chill until mixture begins to thicken. When slightly firm, add drained mandarin orange segments. Turn into 6 small individual molds, and chill until firm.

To serve, unmold on salad plates, and garnish with slices of avocado.

Peaches Pompeii

4 Servings

1 package frozen sliced
  peaches
½ cup syrup from frozen
  peaches

1 package lemon gelatin
1 cup boiling water
½ cup cold water
1 cup applesauce

Thaw the peaches, and drain, keeping ½ cup of the syrup.
Dissolve the gelatin in 1 cup boiling water. Add peach
syrup and ½ cup cold water. Cool until gelatin begins to
thicken. Add peach slices and applesauce.

Spoon mixture into a square baking dish or a medium-size
ring mold, and chill until firm—about 3 to 4 hours. Unmold.
If you are using a baking dish, we suggest cutting the jellied
salad into squares before serving.

Pineapple Ring

8 to 10 Servings

1 package lime gelatin
3 cups boiling water
½ cup crushed pineapple,
  drained

1 package lemon gelatin
1 package (3 ounces) cream
  cheese
1 cup heavy cream, whipped

Dissolve lime gelatin in 1½ cups boiling water, and chill
until it begins to thicken. Fold in drained pineapple, and
pour into ring mold. Chill until firm.

Meanwhile, dissolve lemon gelatin in remaining 1½ cups
boiling water, and chill until it begins to thicken.

Soften cream cheese by working with a large wooden
spoon, and mix with whipped cream; then blend with lemon
gelatin. Pour into mold on top of firm lime gelatin. Chill for
several hours before unmolding.

Diamond Head Potato Salad

4 Servings

8 small new potatoes, boiled
  and peeled
2 eggs, hard-cooked

1 avocado
1 teaspoon lemon juice
Salt

Slice potatoes thinly. Slice hard-cooked eggs.

Peel avocado, and remove pit. Cut into small pieces, and mash with a silver or stainless-steel fork. Add lemon juice and salt to taste. Put this mixture in a blender, and blend until smooth.

Arrange sliced potatoes on salad plates or salad platter. Add a layer of sliced hard-cooked egg. Top with puréed avocado.

This is an excellent salad to serve with cold sliced chicken or turkey.

Black-and-White Molds

6 Servings

1 package (3 ounces) cream
  cheese
4 teaspoons lemon juice
1½ tablespoons sugar

½ cup heavy cream,
  whipped
1½ cups cooked prunes

Mash cream cheese with a wooden spoon; add lemon juice and sugar, then beat until smooth and fluffy.

Whip cream until stiff, and fold into cheese mixture.

Remove pits from cooked prunes, and force prunes through a sieve.

Rinse 6 small individual molds in cold water, and line with cheese mixture; then fill the center of each mold with prune mixture. Place in freezer compartment of refrigerator for 3 to 4 hours. Unmold, and serve immediately.

This salad is a refreshing companion for broiled or roasted chicken.

Use-Up-the-Leftovers Salad

6 Servings

1 cup cooked turkey or
   chicken, diced
1 cup cooked rice
1 cup cooked green beans
Salt

½ cup olive oil
3 tablespoons lemon juice
2 eggs, hard-cooked and
   finely chopped

Combine diced poultry, rice, and green beans in a large mixing bowl. Add salt to taste, oil, and lemon juice. Toss lightly but well. Chill thoroughly. Before serving, sprinkle chopped hard-cooked egg on top.

Desserts

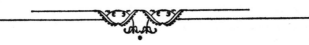

The individual who has been deprived of cigarettes, at least some favorite foods, strong black coffee, and has had to curtail if not eliminate the cocktail hour has a deep need for a feeling of satisfaction at the end of a meal. Eye-catching desserts in small portions fulfill this need.

We feel the ulcer patient will have had his soul tried by puddings and tapiocas by the time you get to this book, so we have concentrated on more spectacular and original desserts. Of course, such popular sweets as pastries, pies, and cakes (except angel food) are taboo. Nuts must not be added to desserts given to an ulcer patient, and chocolate is undesirable too. This does limit the dessert list, but even so we have been able to develop thirty-two recipes.

Throughout our book we have, in many instances, specified the size of the pan or dish a mixture should be put in, and this is especially important in following dessert instructions. The right size dish may not affect the taste, but it has much to do with the appearance of the finished product. Why make a mess when you can make a masterpiece!

Basic Angel Food Cake

Here is one of the few cakes an ulcer patient is allowed to eat.

1 cup sifted cake flour	¼ teaspoon salt
1¼ cups sifted granulated sugar	1 teaspoon cream of tartar
	1 teaspoon vanilla extract
1 cup egg whites (8 to 10 egg whites)	¼ teaspoon almond extract

Sift the flour and ¼ cup of sugar together 4 times.

With an electric beater, beat egg whites and salt until foamy; then add the cream of tartar, and continue beating, at high speed, until the egg whites are stiff and standing in peaks but not dry.

Add the remaining cup of sugar, 2 tablespoons at a time, beating after each addition, until the sugar is blended into the stiff egg whites. Fold in the vanilla and almond extract flavorings.

Sift ¼ cup of the flour-and-sugar mixture over the egg whites, and fold in lightly. Continue doing this, a quarter cup at a time, until all the flour-sugar mixture is used.

Turn into a 9-inch tube pan, and cut through the batter gently with a knife to remove air bubbles. Bake in 325° oven for 1 hour.

Invert cake on a cooling rack for 1 hour before removing from pan.

Apricot Meringues

6 Servings

3 egg whites
1/4 teaspoon salt
1/8 teaspoon cream of tartar
1/4 teaspoon almond extract

1/2 cup sugar
1 can (30 ounces) apricots
1/2 cup heavy cream,
  whipped

Beat egg whites, salt, cream of tartar, and almond extract until foamy. Then beat in the sugar, 1 tablespoon at a time, until the meringue stands in stiff peaks.

With a large spoon, drop the meringue mixture in rounded spoonfuls onto a foil-lined cookie sheet. Bake in a very slow 225° oven for 1 hour. Turn off heat, but leave meringues in the oven for 1 hour longer. Cool on a wire rack, and store in a tightly covered container.

To serve, drain apricots, and purée in blender. Beat heavy cream until stiff. Cover meringues with apricot purée, then top with whipped cream.

Prune-Whip Soufflé

4 Servings

2 jars baby-pack strained
  prunes
1/4 cup sugar
Dash of salt

1 teaspoon lemon juice
3 egg whites
Lemon Sauce (page 201)

Combine prunes, sugar, salt, and lemon juice in a saucepan. Bring to boil; reduce heat, and simmer for 10 minutes. Remove from heat and cool.

Beat egg whites with an electric beater until stiff but not dry. Fold into cooled prune mixture. Spoon mixture into a buttered 1½-quart baking dish, and set baking dish in a pan of hot water. Bake in a 350° oven for 30 minutes.

Serve warm with Lemon Sauce.

Steamed Peach Soufflé

4 Servings

1 jar junior-pack chopped
  peaches
½ cup sugar
Grated rind of ½ lemon

1 tablespoon lemon juice
4 egg whites
¼ teaspoon cream of tartar
Salt

Put peaches, ¼ cup of the sugar, the lemon rind, and lemon juice in a saucepan, and heat just long enough to dissolve sugar, stirring from time to time.

Put egg whites, cream of tartar, and a dash of salt in a mixing bowl. Add the remaining ¼ cup sugar—1 tablespoon at a time—beating very well after each addition. Continue to beat, until egg whites are very stiff, and form peaks. Fold into peach mixture.

Now spoon this mixture into the top of a 2-quart double boiler that has a tight-fitting cover (the cover *must* fit tightly), and place over hot water. Steam, keeping water in the bottom pan just below boiling, for 1 hour. Do *not* remove the cover while soufflé is cooking. Serve warm.

Mousse El Exigente

6 Servings

1½ envelopes unflavored
  gelatin
2 cups water
1 cup milk
¾ cup sugar
¼ teaspoon salt

2 tablespoons instant
  decaffeinated coffee
3 eggs, separated
1 teaspoon vanilla extract
1 cup heavy cream,
  whipped

Soften gelatin in ½ cup cold water.

Mix remaining 1½ cups water with milk, sugar, salt, and instant coffee; pour into the top of a double boiler. Add softened gelatin, and heat until mixture is very hot and gelatin is dissolved, stirring constantly.

Separate eggs, and beat yolks slightly. Add to gelatin mixture. Cook until mixture coats a spoon, stirring constantly. Remove custard from heat, add vanilla, and chill until somewhat thickened.

Meanwhile, beat egg whites until they are stiff but not dry. When custard has cooled, fold in the egg whites. Spoon into individual sherbert glasses, or your prettiest serving bowl, and chill until firm. Serve with whipped cream.

Apricot and Rice Pudding

6 to 8 Servings

2 cups cooked rice
  (do not use packaged
  precooked rice)
1 can (30 ounces) apricot
  halves

Juice from apricot can
1¼ teaspoons unflavored
  gelatin
1 cup heavy cream, whipped
Salt

Cook rice according to directions on box for 2 cups cooked rice, but cook 5 to 10 minutes longer than directed. The rice must be very soft. Do *not* use packaged precooked rice for this recipe. Cool rice to room temperature.

Take 7 apricot halves from can, and drain on a paper towel. Place them in the bottom of a 1-quart soufflé dish.

Apricots should be placed with the rounded side down, as this dessert is to be unmolded.

Put remaining apricots and 2 tablespoons of juice in a blender, and purée. Save remaining juice.

Soften gelatin in 3 tablespoons apricot juice, then dissolve in the top of a double boiler. While gelatin is dissolving, whip cream until stiff.

In a large mixing bowl, combine rice, *puréed* apricots, dissolved gelatin, and a pinch of salt. Mix well. Fold in ¾ cup whipped cream, and spoon into soufflé dish on top of apricot halves. Chill. When firm—about 3 hours—unmold and garnish with remaining whipped cream.

Danish Rice

4 Servings

1 cup packaged precooked rice
1½ cups milk
¼ cup sugar
¼ teaspoon salt

1 teaspoon vanilla extract
1 jar junior-pack strained apricots or peaches
¾ cup heavy cream, whipped

Combine rice, milk, sugar, and salt. Cook according to directions on rice box. Remove from heat, and let stand for 15 minutes. (Mixture will be thin.) Add vanilla extract; cover, and cool in refrigerator.

When mixture is slightly chilled, fold in one jar of strained apricots or peaches. Whip cream, and fold into rice and fruit. Pour into 4 custard cups or dessert dishes, and chill.

Caramel Riz Gâteau

6 Servings

1½ cups rice (do not use
   packaged precooked rice)
4 cups milk
1 teaspoon vanilla extract
4 egg yolks

4 tablespoons butter, melted
⅔ cup sugar, plus ½ cup
   sugar
Whipped cream for garnish

Cook rice for 3 minutes only, following directions on box for proper amount of water. Drain, and mix rice with milk and vanilla extract. Place in a buttered baking dish, and bake, covered, in 375° oven for 45 minutes to 1 hour. *Do not stir.* Rice should be almost dry when removed from oven.

Beat egg yolks until they are light and frothy. Melt butter in the top of a small double boiler. Stir butter into beaten eggs. Add ⅔ cup sugar, and mix well.

Add the rice to the eggs, butter, and sugar mixture, and stir thoroughly, breaking up the rice grains as much as possible. Set aside.

Now, melt ½ cup sugar in a 9½ x 5½ x 2½-inch cake pan over *very low heat,* until the sugar has dissolved and turns a golden caramel color. Tilt the pan constantly to coat the bottom and sides thoroughly with syrup. Spoon rice mixture into caramel-coated pan. Set cake pan in a larger pan half-filled with hot water, and bake in 375° oven for 30 minutes.

Cool rice cake in pan. When cool, unmold on serving platter and garnish with whipped cream, if desired.

The Senator's Rice Pudding

6 Servings

2 eggs, beaten
1½ cups milk
Dash of salt
4 tablespoons butter, melted
1 teaspoon lemon juice

1 teaspoon vanilla extract
2 cups cooked rice
   (do not use packaged
  precooked rice)

Beat the eggs well, and add the milk, salt, butter, lemon juice, and vanilla, beating all the while. Now mix in the cooked rice with a light hand. Spoon mixture into a medium-size buttered baking dish.

Bake in 325° oven for about 45 minutes, until the pudding has set. This dish may be served either hot or cold, and you can garnish with whipped cream if you wish.

After spooning out one portion for the ulcer patient, you can add ½ cup raisins and ½ cup finely chopped almonds to the remaining pudding for the other members of the family.

Lemon Rice Puffs

6 Servings

¼ cup butter
½ cup sugar
1 teaspoon grated lemon
  rind
3 eggs, separated

3 tablespoons lemon juice
1½ cups milk
¾ cup packaged precooked
  rice

Cream butter, sugar, and lemon rind together until light and fluffy. Beat egg yolks, and fold in. Add lemon juice, milk, and rice. (Mixture will look curdled.)

Beat egg whites until stiff, and fold into rice mixture. Pour into 6 lightly buttered custard cups. Set cups in a shallow pan, and pour hot water around cups to ½-inch depth. Bake in 350° oven for 30 minutes. Serve warm.

Crunchy Apples

4 Servings

¼ cup water	⅓ cup quick-cooking oats
½ teaspoon grated lemon rind	3 tablespoons flour
⅔ cup sugar	3 tablespoons brown sugar
2 apples, peeled, cored, and halved	2 tablespoons butter, melted
	½ cup heavy cream, whipped

Combine water, lemon rind, and sugar in a small saucepan, and heat to boiling. Place apple halves in pan, cover, and simmer for 10 minutes or until apples are tender but still firm enough to hold their shape.

Lift apples from syrup and place, cut-side up, in an 8-inch pie plate. Pour syrup over apples.

Combine the oats, flour, and brown sugar in a small bowl. Stir in butter until the mixture is crumbly. Pat evenly over apple halves. Bake in 400° oven for 20 minutes, or until top is brown. Spoon into dessert dishes, and top with whipped cream. Serve warm.

Banana Caribbean

4 Servings

2 tablespoons butter
½ teaspoon rum
¼ cup honey

4 medium-size bananas,
    peeled
2 teaspoons grated orange
    rind

Melt butter in the top of a large double boiler. Stir in rum and honey. Place bananas in syrup mixture and heat, turning once, for about 15 minutes, or until lightly glazed.

Place bananas on dessert plates, and spoon sauce over the tops. Sprinkle with grated orange rind, and serve warm.

Banana Honey

4 Servings

4 bananas, peeled
4 tablespoons orange juice

3 tablespoons unsweetened
    pineapple juice
¼ cup honey

Cut bananas into small rounds, and place in a 1-quart baking dish that has a cover.

Combine fruit juices and honey, and pour over bananas. Bake in a 350° oven for 10 minutes; uncover, and bake 5 minutes longer, or until bananas are tender. Serve warm.

Southern Banana Bake

4 Servings

2 large, firm bananas
1 cup heavy cream

2 tablespoons brown sugar

Peel bananas, and cut into rounds. Put into 4 individual 3½-inch custard ramekins. Pour ¼ cup heavy cream over banana in each ramekin. Sprinkle with brown sugar—½ teaspoon to each ramekin.

Bake in 350° oven for 30 minutes. (Put a baking sheet or foil on the lower shelf of the oven, as this dish bubbles.) Serve warm.

Cerises au Vin

8 Servings

2 cans (14 ounces each) dark, pitted cherries
Juice from cherries
2 cups water
1¼ cups red wine, claret preferred

Thinly peeled rinds from ½ lemon and ½ orange
Salt
2 tablespoons tapioca, the quick-cooking type

Drain cherries, reserving juice; force cherries through a sieve.

Combine cherry purée, cherry juice, water, wine, fruit rinds, and salt to taste in a saucepan, cooking slowly for about 10 minutes.

Strain into another pan, and bring back to a boil. Add tapioca, cooking slowly for another 10 minutes.

Chill thoroughly before serving.

Orange Igloos

6 Servings

6 *large* oranges	3 egg whites
½ cup grenadine syrup	½ cup sugar
Cointreau (a few drops)	1 pint vanilla ice cream

Several hours before serving, cut the tops off oranges, and scoop out pulp. Remove seeds, place orange pulp in a bowl, and pour on grenadine mixed with a drop or two of Cointreau. Let stand. Turn scooped-out orange shells upside down in a shallow bowl to drain.

To finish dessert: Preheat oven to 400°. Beat egg whites until stiff but not dry. Add ½ cup sugar, gradually, beating until meringue is glossy and stiff.

Turn drained orange shells right-side up. Fill with a little vanilla ice cream, then a layer of orange pulp, then another small layer of ice cream. Fill remaining space in orange shells with meringue, and mound on top in rounded peaks. Bake for 8 to 10 minutes, or until golden brown.

Honolulu Peaches

4 Servings

4 large, firm fresh peaches	¼ cup canned, unsweetened
¼ cup sugar	pineapple juice

Peel peaches by pouring boiling water over them, and lightly rubbing off the skins. Place peaches close together in a baking dish that has a cover. Sprinkle with sugar, pour pineapple juice over all. Cover, and bake in 350° oven for 25 minutes. Remove cover, and brown fruit lightly by leaving in oven for 5 to 10 minutes longer. Serve warm.

Baked Pears

4 Servings

4 large pears
4 tablespoons brown sugar
⅓ cup water

2 tablespoons butter
Grated rind of ½ a lemon
Devonshire Illusion Sauce (page 200)

Wash and peel pears. Set aside.

Combine brown sugar, water, and butter in a small saucepan. Bring syrup to boil, and pour over pears that have been placed upright in a deep baking dish that has a cover. Trim bottoms of pears if necessary, so they will stand upright. Sprinkle with grated lemon rind.

Cover and bake in 375° oven for 1 hour, basting pears occasionally. Serve hot with Devonshire Illusion Sauce.

Pineapple Loaf

4 Servings

½ cup butter
1½ cups confectioners' sugar
2 eggs, separated
½ teaspoon lemon extract

¾ cup canned crushed pineapple, drained
1 cup commercial sour cream

Cream the butter and sugar until fluffy. Add the egg yolks, one at a time, beating well each time. Stir in lemon extract and crushed pineapple.

Beat egg whites until stiff but not dry.

Fold sour cream into pineapple mixture, then fold in egg whites. Spoon the mixture into a loaf pan, about 8 x 4 x 2 inches, and chill for 6 to 8 hours before serving.

Plum Dandy

8 Servings

2 pounds red plums
  (about 10)
2 medium-size tart apples
2 cups sugar

½ cup flour
½ cup honey
2 tablespoons butter, melted
Vanilla ice cream

Halve plums, pit, and cut into thin slices. Pare apples, core, and slice thinly.

Combine plums and apples, and put in a lightly buttered baking dish that has a lid. Sprinkle with sugar and flour, then pour on honey and melted butter. Cover, and bake in 400° oven for 30 minutes.

Serve warm with scoops of vanilla ice cream.

Fruits Helène

4 Servings

1 can (8¾ ounces) sliced
  cling peaches
1 can (8¾ ounces) dark
  cherries, pitted

1 can (8¾ ounces) Bartlett
  pears
1 banana
Vanilla-Rum Sauce (page
  202)

Empty fruits, including juices, into a saucepan. Peel and slice banana, and add.

Place pan, *covered,* on very low flame, and heat. Be sure you neither boil nor simmer fruit, just heat. Serve when warm but not really hot.

This compote is delicious with Vanilla-Rum Sauce.

Classic Fruit Gelatin

8 Servings

1 package lemon gelatin
1 cup boiling water
1 can (16 ounces) tropical
  fruit salad or fruit
  cocktail

1 jar (16 ounces) citrus fruit
  salad
1 cup juice from canned
  fruits

Dissolve gelatin in 1 cup boiling water in a large mixing bowl.

Drain fruits, reserving can juices. Add 1 cup can juice to the gelatin, and stir to mix. (Do *not* add fruits at this time.) Pour into a mold that has been rinsed in cold water, and chill until gelatin is slightly thick and beginning to set.

Then stir in fruits, and return to refrigerator. Chill until firm before unmolding.

Homemade Banana Ice Cream

4 Servings

4 ripe bananas, peeled
4 teaspoons lemon juice

8 tablespoons heavy cream
4 tablespoons sugar

Halve peeled bananas and mash pulp somewhat with a fork. Combine all ingredients in a blender. Blend for 5 seconds until mixture is creamy.

Spoon into individual serving bowls or one large container, and place in freezer for 2 to 3 hours, until mixture reaches the consistency of ice cream.

If you leave mixture in the freezer for only one hour, it

makes a cream that is delectable served over drained, canned fruits.

Should your blender not hold the amounts suggested above, halve the ingredients and run blender twice.

Roman Parfait

6 Servings

⅔ cup sugar   Salt
¼ cup water   1 cup heavy cream, whipped
2 egg whites   2 tablespoons vanilla extract

Cook sugar and water in a small saucepan, stirring constantly, until mixture spins a thread when dripped from a spoon.

Meanwhile beat egg whites with a pinch of salt until they are stiff. Slowly pour the sugar-and-water syrup, a little at a time, into stiff egg whites, beating constantly. Cool.

Whip cream, add vanilla. When egg-white mixture is cool, fold in whipped cream. Spoon into parfait glasses, and freeze until firm.

Crème Brulée Facile

4 to 6 Servings

The first part of this recipe should be prepared the day before serving.

1 package vanilla-pudding   ½ cup light-brown sugar,
    mix   packed tightly in
1½ cups milk   measuring cup
1½ cups heavy cream

On the day before, make vanilla pudding following directions on the package label, but substituting 1½ cups milk and 1½ cups heavy cream for the 2 cups of milk the package label calls for. Pour into 1½-quart baking dish, then put a piece of aluminum foil directly on the surface of the pudding. Refrigerate.

An hour or so before dessert time, preheat broiler for 10 minutes. Remove foil from pudding and sift brown sugar over top. Put baking dish on broiler rack, about 3 inches from heat. Broil just until sugar melts, making a caramel top. Refrigerate until time to serve.

Maple Cream

8 *Servings*

1 package vanilla-pudding mix	½ cup maple syrup
1 envelope unflavored gelatin	3 eggs, separated
	¼ teaspoon cream of tartar
1⅓ cups water	½ cup sugar
	1 cup heavy cream, whipped

Combine pudding mix and gelatin in a medium-size saucepan; stir in ⅓ cup water and maple syrup. Beat in egg yolks, then stir in remaining 1 cup water.

Cook slowly, stirring constantly, until mixture thickens and starts to bubble. Pour into a large bowl, and press a sheet of foil directly on surface of the pudding. Chill for about 1½ hours.

While mixture chills, beat egg whites with cream of tartar until stiff. Beat in sugar, 1 tablespoon at a time, until meringue is peaky.

Whip cream until stiff.

When pudding mixture has cooled, fold in meringue; then fold in *half* the whipped cream, until no white streaks remain. Spoon into a large serving bowl, and chill several hours until firm. Garnish with remaining whipped cream.

Custard with Meringues

4 eggs	Salt
6 tablespoons sugar *plus*	2 cups milk
½ cup sugar	¼ teaspoon vanilla extract

Separate eggs; beat yolks until thick and lemon-colored. Blend in 6 tablespoons sugar and a dash of salt. Set aside.

Beat egg whites with an electric beater until stiff but not dry. Add ½ cup sugar gradually, beating all the while. Set meringue mixture aside.

Heat milk to scalding in the top of a large, wide double boiler. Drop meringue mixture by tablespoonfuls on top of the scalding milk. Cook for 3 minutes until meringues are firm. Lift out meringues with a large perforated spoon and set aside. Reduce heat under double boiler as soon as meringues have been removed.

Now stir ½ cup scalded milk slowly into egg yolk and sugar mixture, then pour back into remaining milk. Cook, stirring constantly, over *low* heat (water in the bottom of double boiler should *not* boil) for 15 to 20 minutes, or until custard thickens slightly and coats a spoon. (Custard will be thin.)

Remove from heat and add vanilla. Pour into a shallow, medium-size dessert bowl and chill. After custard has cooled for 15 minutes, remove from refrigerator and float meringues on top. Return to refrigerator and chill thoroughly before serving.

Cheese Custard Hollande

4 to 6 Servings

1 cup large-curd creamed
 cottage cheese
1 cup cream
½ cup confectioners' sugar

¼ teaspoon salt
5 eggs, separated
4 tablespoons butter, melted

Push cottage cheese through a fine sieve into a mixing bowl. Stir in cream, sugar, salt, beaten egg yolks, and melted butter.

Beat the egg whites until stiff; fold into cheese mixture.

Lightly butter a 9-inch pie pan, and pour in the cheese custard. Bake in 450° oven for 10 minutes. Reduce heat to 350°, and bake for another 20 minutes. Cool before serving.

Moroccan Custard

4 Servings

2 eggs
3 tablespoons sugar
Salt
1½ cups milk

2 teaspoons instant decaffeinated coffee
¼ teaspoon vanilla extract

Beat eggs slightly with sugar and a dash of salt. Stir in milk, instant coffee, and vanilla. Mix very well, and pour into 4 custard cups.

Pour 1 inch of boiling water into a shallow baking pan. Set cups in pan and bake in 325° oven for 40 minutes, or until centers are almost set but still soft. (Do not overbake, as custard will set as it cools.) Remove cups from water at once, and cool.

Heavenly Banana Pudding

6 to 8 Servings

1 package vanilla-pudding
  mix
1 cup heavy cream, whipped
1½ cups miniature
  marshmallows

2 bananas, sliced
1 cup canned mandarin-
  orange segments, drained

Prepare pudding mix according to directions on package,
and cool.

Whip cream and set aside.

When pudding has cooled, fold in whipped cream, marshmallows, bananas, and ½ cup of mandarin-orange segments.
Pour into individual sherbet dishes, and chill until ready
to serve.

Garnish with remaining ½ cup of mandarin-orange segments.

Normandy Pudding

4 to 6 Servings

1 box (6 ounces) elbow
  macaroni
3 cups applesauce
½ cup sugar

2 tablespoons lemon juice
4 tablespoons butter
3 tablespoons breadcrumbs

Cook macaroni according to directions on box. Drain,
and rinse with a dash of cold water.

In a large buttered baking dish, put a layer of cooked macaroni. Mix applesauce with sugar and lemon juice. Spread 2 cups applesauce mixture on top of macaroni. Dot with 2 tablespoons butter. Cover with the remaining macaroni, spread with 1 cup applesauce mixture, and dot with 1 tablespoon butter. Sprinkle top with breadcrumbs, and dot with remaining 1 tablespoon butter. Bake in 350° oven for 20 minutes. Serve warm.

Tapioca el Hombre

4 Servings

3 tablespoons quick-cooking tapioca
⅓ cup sugar
3 teaspoons instant decaffeinated coffee
1 egg, beaten

1½ cups milk
Salt
½ teaspoon vanilla extract
½ cup heavy cream, whipped

Mix tapioca, sugar, instant coffee, lightly beaten egg, milk, and a dash of salt in a medium-size saucepan. Let stand for 5 minutes.

Heat slowly to a rolling boil, stirring constantly. Remove from heat immediately, and cool. Stir in vanilla. Chill.

When ready to serve, spoon the mixture, alternating with whipped cream, into 4 parfait glasses.

Sauces

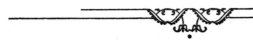

A beautiful sauce adds interest and character to many innocuous dishes, but this is a difficult area for the one who is preparing food for an ulcer patient. To go right to the heart of the matter, the cook must always remember that fat—butter or margarine—and flour should *never* be put in a pan that is placed directly over heat. The sensitive stomach cannot cope with flour that has been browned in fat. Fortunately, digestible sauces can be made in the top of a double boiler; most fine cooks use this technique, so it is well worth learning.

For thickening a too watery stew, use our European method of adding small amounts of flour to a sauce, page 197. Condensed soups can be used as sauces or in casserole cooking, but be certain to avoid soups containing onions and spices.

Whenever possible, use one of the new instant-blending flour products in making sauces. This type of flour blends instantly in cold or hot water.

Delicious fruit sauces for desserts may be made very easily by draining a can of apricots or peaches, for example, putting the fruit in your blender, and puréeing for a few minutes. Add a little of the juice from the can if the sauce needs thinning.

European Sauce Thickening Method

If you are not using an instant-blending flour product, this is the proper way to add a thickening agent to a sauce or gravy for an ulcer-diet patient:

Fill a jelly jar, or other small jar that has a screw top, about ½ to ¾ full with *warm* tap water. Add 1 tablespoon all-purpose flour (depending on how thick you want the sauce) to the warm water. Close the jar, and shake vigorously until all flour is dissolved and no lumps remain. The secret is in using *warm* water.

Our Mandalay House Mayonnaise

1 Cup

1 egg
2 tablespoons lemon juice

¼ teaspoon salt
1 cup olive oil

Put egg, lemon juice, salt, and only ¼ cup oil in blender. Cover, and blend for 12 seconds. Remove cover, and, with blender still running, pour in the rest of the oil in a steady stream. Stop blender as soon as last bit of oil is poured in.

Blender Hollandaise

¾ Cup

½ cup butter, melted
2 egg yolks

1 tablespoon fresh lemon
  juice
¼ teaspoon salt

Melt the butter in the top of a small double boiler. Heat until butter is very hot and bubbly.

Put egg yolks, lemon juice, and salt in a blender, and blend for a few seconds. While blender is going, slowly pour in melted butter. Stop blender as soon as last bit of butter has been poured in.

Our Hollandaise can be kept warm in the top of a double boiler, but boiling water must not touch upper pan.

Sauce Verte

2 Cups

¼ cup junior-pack chopped
  spinach
1 can cream of celery soup,
  (undiluted)

1 cup milk
1 tablespoon fresh lemon
  juice

Combine all ingredients in a blender, and blend just until smooth. Pour into a small saucepan, and heat over low fire until sauce is thoroughly heated. This sauce is meant to be served hot, and is very good with fish or chicken.

Quick Spinach Sauce

About 1½ Cups

1 package frozen creamed
spinach (in immersible
plastic bag)

2 to 3 tablespoons milk

Prepare spinach in its plastic bag according to directions. When thoroughly heated, remove from bag, and thin with 2 to 3 tablespoons milk. Reheat for a minute, if necessary.

This is a good and quick sauce to serve with noodles or with Daffodil Eggs, page 150.

Sour Cream Sauce

1 Cup

1 cup commercial sour cream
Yolk of hard-cooked egg

2 tablespoons butter
Salt

Put sour cream into a small mixing bowl. Press the yolk of hard-cooked egg through a fine sieve, and add to sour cream. Blend well.

Pour mixture into the top of a double boiler; add butter and salt to taste.

Heat thoroughly, and serve over cooked vegetables.

Taste of Honey Dressing

About 1½ Cups

1 cup commercial sour cream
½ cup honey

Juice of 1 lemon
Salt to taste

Combine all ingredients, and mix very well. Chill before serving on fruit-salad molds or any salad made with canned fruits.

This dressing will keep for three to four days in the refrigerator if stored in a tightly covered container.

Devonshire Illusion

About 2 Cups

1 package (8 ounces) cream cheese

½ cup commercial sour cream

Soften cream cheese, then beat in sour cream with an electric beater, until the mixture is light and smooth. If necessary, add a bit more sour cream.

Serve this sauce over cooked or canned fruits.

New Orleans Dessert Sauce

1¼ Cups

1 cup commercial sour cream
2 egg yolks
¼ cup sugar

¼ teaspoon salt
2 tablespoons Grand
  Marnier

Combine all ingredients in a blender, and blend for a few seconds. Chill for 1 hour.

This is an excellent sauce for baked peaches or baked apples.

Easy Lemon Sauce

About 1¼ Cups

½ cup sugar
1 tablespoon cornstarch
Salt
1 cup water

1 teaspoon grated lemon
  rind
3 tablespoons lemon juice
1 tablespoon butter

Combine sugar, cornstarch, and salt to taste in a saucepan; pour in water slowly, and stir very well. Cook over medium heat, stirring constantly, until mixture thickens and boils for 1 minute.

Stir in lemon rind, lemon juice, and butter. Mix well. Remove from heat the moment the butter is melted. Chill.

Serve with stewed fruit, bread pudding, or rice pudding.

Strawberry Sauce

About 2 Cups

1 package frozen sliced
strawberries, somewhat
thawed

1 tablespoon sugar
¼ cup water

Combine partly thawed strawberries and their juice with
the sugar and water in a medium-size saucepan. Heat to
boiling, stirring constantly. Reduce heat, and cook for 10
minutes, stirring until slightly thickened. Pour through
fine sieve. Chill.

Serve on vanilla ice cream or vanilla pudding.

Vanilla-Rum Sauce

About 1½ Cups

½ pint heavy cream
1 tablespoon sugar

1 teaspoon vanilla extract
¼ cup rum, or to taste

Whip the cream lightly with the sugar, adding vanilla
extract gradually. Whip just until mixture reaches the consistency of a thick sauce, no more. Add rum and stir very
well. Refrigerate.

Serve with cooked fruits or over ice cream.

Shakes and Other Drinks

Because the number of teenage ulcer victims is on the rise, we are including a few shake recipes to delight the younger as well as the older set. The latter group should, of course, ration their quota of shakes if weight control is a problem.

Canned fruits are your best bet. Fresh fruit can be used in shake combinations for an ulcer sufferer only if the fruit is completely puréed. Remember, fruit skins and seeds must be carefully removed before blending. If you cannot remove the seeds prior to blending, we advise putting the mixture through a fine sieve before serving.

In general, chocolate should not be used in shakes. Many doctors do allow their patients to have cocoa and milk mixtures, but the cocoa should be used solely as a flavoring agent.

Young people tend to gulp drinks, and this is not good for any ulcer patient, teenage or middle-aged. Needless to say, ice-cold drinks should not be given to anyone during an acute digestive upset.

Dreamy Banana Malt

2 to 3 Servings

1 cup milk
1 ripe banana, peeled and
    quartered

1 tablespoon malted milk
    powder
1 large scoop vanilla ice
    cream

Put milk, banana, and malted milk powder in blender. Cover, and blend 10 seconds.

Add ice cream, and cover again. Blend 10 seconds. If ice cream is very hard, blend an additional 5 seconds. Serve in large glasses.

Secret Ingredient Banana Frosty

2 Servings

1 large ripe banana
1 teaspoon brown sugar
½ cup evaporated milk

½ cup milk
1 cup cracked ice

Peel and cut banana into small pieces. Put all ingredients in a blender, and blend until drink is smooth—about 1 minute. This is a very rich, sweet shake that appeals to little boys and the boy within the man. The secret ingredient in this recipe is the evaporated milk.

Oklahoma Shake

3 Servings

4 tablespoons lemon juice
4 tablespoons sugar

2 cups buttermilk
1 cup cracked ice

Mix lemon juice with sugar and stir until well mixed. Pour buttermilk into a blender, add sugar and lemon juice mixture, and blend for 30 seconds. Pour over cracked ice, and serve immediately.

Cherry Float

6 Servings

1 envelope unsweetened, cherry-flavored, soft-drink powder

1 cup sugar
2 cups milk
1 quart vanilla ice cream

Put the soft-drink powder, sugar, and milk in a bowl. Stir until completely dissolved. Pour into 6 large glasses. Add scoops of ice cream to each glass, and stir to muddle a little.

Coffee-Flavor Float

4 Servings

¼ cup instant decaffeinated
coffee
2 tablespoons sugar

3 cups water
1 pint vanilla ice cream
½ cup heavy cream, whipped

Combine the coffee powder, sugar, and water in a saucepan. Cover, and bring to a boil. Remove from heat and let stand, covered, 5 minutes to steep. Chill well.

Meanwhile, chill 4 tall glasses, and pour about ⅓ cup of the cold coffee mixture into each. Add several tablespoonfuls of ice cream, stirring to mix slightly. Add the remaining coffee mix, and top with a dollop of whipped cream.

Tall, Tan, and Terrific

3 Servings

1½ cups milk
1 heaping tablespoon instant
decaffeinated coffee
1 heaping tablespoon instant
cocoa or cocoa mix

1 teaspoon almond extract
1 tablespoon brown sugar
1 cup cracked ice

Combine all ingredients in a blender, and whirl at high speed for 1 minute. Pour into tall glasses. This is a frothy-light, non-sweet shake that many men find appealing.

Maple Milk Shake

2 Servings

2 cups milk
4 tablespoons maple syrup

Cracked ice, if desired

Put milk and maple syrup in blender, and blend until light and frothy. Add cracked ice, if desired, and serve in tall glasses.

Canario

2 Servings

1 cup milk
½ cup orange juice
1 cup cracked ice

1 tablespoon lemon juice
1 tablespoon sugar

Put all ingredients in a blender and turn to high speed. Blend thoroughly about 30 seconds. Serve in tall glasses.

Pineapple Blossom

2 Servings

1 cup milk
1 cup canned crushed
  pineapple

½ teaspoon vanilla
1 tablespoon sugar
1 cup cracked ice

Place all ingredients in a blender, and blend at high speed until contents are thoroughly mixed—about 1 minute. Serve in tall glasses.

Strawberry Milk Shake

4 Servings

1 pint vanilla ice cream
3 cups milk

½ cup strawberry *jelly*
Whipped cream for garnish

Combine all ingredients except whipped cream in blender, and blend well. Pour into tall glasses, and garnish with whipped cream and a dollop of jelly. Do not use strawberry *jam,* because of the seeds.

Superfruit Frosty

3 Servings

½ cup grape juice
½ cup pineapple juice
½ cup apricot nectar

½ cup orange juice
2 tablespoons sugar
1 cup cracked ice

Place all ingredients in your blender, and blend at high speed until all flavors are thoroughly mixed—about 15 seconds.

Holiday Eggnog

8 Servings

2 eggs, separated
¼ cup sugar
2 cups milk
2 tablespoons rum

½ teaspoon vanilla
Salt
1 cup heavy cream

Beat egg whites until stiff. Beat in 2 tablespoons of sugar, a tablespoon at a time, continuing to beat until the meringue stands in firm peaks.

Beat the 2 egg yolks until foamy and lemon-colored. Beat in remaining sugar; pour in the milk, rum, vanilla, and a pinch of salt. Pour mixture into a blender, and whirl for a few seconds.

Beat cream until stiff.

Pour egg and milk mixture into a large bowl, fold in the meringue, then fold in the whipped cream, saving ½ cup of whipped cream to mound on top.

The Long-Face Lifter

5 Servings

This is not a shake, but we are including this cooler for those ulcer patients who formerly enjoyed the pleasures of the glass. Served on a hot summer evening, this beverage makes an agreeable substitute for gin and tonic or Tom Collins.

1 cup water
½ cup sugar
Grated rind of 1 orange
2 cups orange juice

3 tablespoons lemon juice
2 cups cold, weak tea
Orange slices for garnish, if desired

Boil water, sugar, and orange rind for five minutes. Strain to remove orange rind, and chill sugar and water mixture. When cool, add fruit juices and tea. Refrigerate until ready to serve. Pour into a pitcher half filled with ice. Garnish with orange slices, if desired.

Canapés

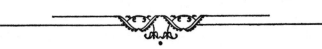

Why are we including a chapter on canapés when alcohol is one of the first things an ulcer patient is told to give up? After much careful thought and questioning of ulcer graduates, we have decided to devote some space to this category of food for the simple reason that most individuals with healed ulcers *do* drink cocktails. The doctor may not approve, nor do the authors of this book. But, in trying to make this a practical guide to ulcer-diet cooking, we feel it is better to face the reality of the cocktail hour. With this in mind, we can only suggest that if the patient is going to drink, he will be far better off not doing it on an empty stomach.

In the canapé category the ulcer patient is severely limited. Most snack foods are either highly seasoned, or contain onions. Nuts are forbidden; potato chips and corn chips, popcorn, sharp cheese, most smoked fish, cocktail frank-furters, and shrimp are not allowed.

The few recipes for canapés and dips that appear in this book contain none of the above ingredients, but are tasty enough so you need not be reluctant to serve them to guests. More important, whether or not he is imbibing, psychologically they help the patient to preserve the illusion and warm camaraderie of the cocktail hour.

Cocktail Feuille Artichaut

4 to 6 Servings

2 artichokes
1 can (7 ounces) tuna **in**
water pack, drained

4 tablespoons our
mayonnaise (page 197)

Cook 2 artichokes. (See page 117 for simple and reliable instructions.) Cool. Remove the leaves one by one; set aside the small outer leaves and also the soft inner leaves and hearts. Save these for another occasion. Put only the large firm leaves on a serving platter, hollow side up.

Blend the drained tuna with the mayonnaise to make a fairly firm mixture. Put a small teaspoonful of this mixture on the fleshy end of each leaf and let your guests help themselves.

Remember to have napkins and extra plates handy for discarded leaves.

Avocado Dip

About 1¼ Cups

2 packages (3 ounces each)
cream cheese
3 tablespoons cream

1 ripe avocado
1 teaspoon lemon juice
Salt to taste

Soften cream cheese by working with a large wooden spoon; add cream and blend well.

Peel avocado, remove pit, and mash pulp with a silver or stainless-steel fork. Put *all* ingredients in a blender, and blend until completely smooth.

Spread on water biscuits.

Acapulco Cocktail Spread

About 2 Cups

2 large ripe avocados, pitted
and peeled
1 can (7 ounces) tuna, in
water pack, drained

2½ tablespoons lemon juice
Salt

Mash the avocados with a silver or stainless-steel fork, and combine with the drained tuna, lemon juice, and salt to taste. Mix well, cover tightly, and chill until ready to serve. Spread on water biscuits or unsalted crackers.

Aztec Spread

6 Servings

2 ripe avocados, pitted and
peeled
2 teaspoons lemon juice

Salt
2 egg whites, beaten stiff
¼ cup heavy cream, whipped

Mash avocado meat with a silver or stainless-steel fork, and force through a fine sieve. Add lemon juice and salt to taste; blend well.

Beat egg whites until stiff but not dry. Whip cream until stiff. Fold egg whites, a little at a time, into avocado mixture; then fold in whipped cream. Chill.

Serve with plain crackers.

Gold Fingers

4 Servings

6 slices day-old bread
1 cup grated mild American cheese

2 tablespoons heavy cream
2 tablespoons sherry
Salt

Remove crusts from bread, and cut each piece into 4 finger-size slices. Toast under broiler on one side only.

Mix grated cheese, cream, sherry, and a dash of salt into a rough paste. Spread untoasted side of bread-fingers with the mixture, and arrange in a single layer on a cookie sheet. Bake in 450° oven for 6 minutes, or until golden brown.

Chicken Dip

2 Cups

2 cups leftover chicken, diced into very small pieces
1 container (12 ounces) cottage cheese (*not* creamed cottage cheese)

¼ cup our mayonnaise (page 197)
Salt to taste
2 tablespoons dry sherry

Put all ingredients into a blender, and let it go. When mixture is completely smooth, pile into a bowl, and chill. Serve with white toast triangles.

Different Deviled Eggs

12 Egg Halves

6 eggs, hard-cooked
1 package (3 ounces) cream
 cheese

Juice of ½ a lemon
4 tablespoons olive oil
Salt to taste

Cut eggs in half, and remove yolks. Mash yolks, and mix with all other ingredients, blending until very smooth. Refill the white halves with mixture, topping well. Chill.

Foie Gras Illusion

2 Cups

Most commercial patés will be too spicy for your patient, but he or she should have no trouble digesting this foie gras.

½ lb. chicken livers, broiled
 and chopped (Do not
 broil too long; chicken
 livers should *not* have
 hard-cooked edges.)

1 package (3 ounces) cream
 cheese, softened
1 tablespoon butter, melted
Salt to taste
1 tablespoon sherry

Put chopped chicken livers and softened cream cheese into a blender. Add all other ingredients, and blend for 1 minute. Chill before serving on dry, thin toast.

Sardine Paté Canapés

Spread for 10 water biscuits

2 cans small sardines (*not* tomato packed)
4 tablespoons butter, softened

2 eggs, hard-cooked and sliced
Water biscuits

Drain the sardines very well, and mash with a fork. Add softened butter, and continue mixing until you get a smooth paste. Chill just slightly.

This paté should not be served too cold. To serve, spread paste on water biscuits, and top with a slice of hard-cooked egg.

Index

Acapulco Cocktail Spread, 213
Acorn Squash, Honey-Baked, 130
Alpine Appetizer, 27
American Soufflé, 154–155
Angel Food Cake, Basic, 174
Appetizer(s), 21–29
  Alpine, 27
  Artichokes à la Moscow, 22
  Avocado Mousse, 23
  Avocado Varié, 24
  Céleri-Rave Hors d'Oeuvre, 24–25
  Chicken-Avocado, 26
  Chicken-Citron Mousse, 26–27
  Chicken Custard, 25
  First-Course Stuffed Tomatoes, 28–29
  Gazpacho Aspic, 28
  Open Apple Rarebit, 22
Apple Rarebit, Open, 22
Apple-Yam Dandy, 111
Apples, Crunchy, 181
Apricot Meringues, 175
Apricot and Rice Pudding, 177–178
Arroz Redondo, 142
Artichaut, Cocktail Feuille, 212
Artichokes, directions for cooking, 117
Artichokes à la Moscow, 22
Artichokes à la Sidney, 118
Artichokes Saint Germain, 117–118
Asparagus in Celery Jelly, 161
Asparagus Eggs, Frothy, 152–153
Asparagus Jockey Club, 162

Asparagus, Scalloped, and Egg Casserole, 119
Asparagus with Summer Squash, 118–119
Avocado-Chicken Appetizer, 26
Avocado Cocktail Spread (Acapulco), 213
Avocado Dip, 212
Avocado Mousse, 23
Avocado Soup, 33
Avocado Spread (Aztec), 213
Avocado Varié, 24
Aztec Spread, 213

Baked Chicken, Beaumont, 74
Baked Chicken, Sidney's, 76
Baked Halibut au Gratin, 92
Baked Omelet, 149
Baked Pears, 185
Baked Ravioli, 140–141
Banana Bake, Southern, 183
Banana Caribbean, 182
Banana Frosty, 204
Banana Honey, 182
Banana Ice Cream, 187–188
Banana Malt, Dreamy, 204
Banana Pudding, Heavenly, 192
Basic Angel Food Cake, 174
Basic Boeuf Bourguignon, 48–49
Beaumont Chicken Bake, 74
Beef, Bohemian, 45
Beef, Flamingo, 56
Beef, Minsk, 49
Beef, Viennese Boiled, 48
Beef-Noodle Casserole, 55
Beets à la Crème, 120

Beets, Orange-Buttered, 120
Black-and-White Molds, 170–171
Blender Hollandaise, 198
Boeuf Bourguignon, 48–49
Boeuf en Gelée, 46–47
Bohemian Beef, 45
Boiled Tomato Tongue, 66
Boneless Red Snapper, 96
Borscht in a Minute, 33
Braised Endives, 126–127
Broccoli, Tomato Stuffed with, 133
Broiled Calf's Liver au Citron, 66
Broiled Chicken, Sweet and Low, 70

Cajun Rice, 145
Cake
    Angel Food, 174
    Caramel Riz Gâteau, 179
Calf's Liver au Citron, Broiled, 66
Canapé(s), 211–216
    Acapulco Cocktail Spread, 213
    Avocado Dip, 212
    Aztec Spread, 213
    Chicken Dip, 214
    Cocktail Feuille Artichaut, 212
    Different Deviled Eggs, 215
    Foie Gras Illusion, 215
    Gold Fingers, 214
    Sardine Paté, 216
Canario, 207
Caramel Riz Gâteau, 179
Carrots Glazed with Honey and
        Orange, 121
Carrots Hong Kong, 122
Carrots, The Very Best in the
        Whole World, 121
Carrots Vichy, 122
Casserole(s)
    Beef-Noodle, 55
    Chicken
        Chicken Noodle, 81
        Normandy, 80–81
        Poulet aux Légumes, 72–73
    Chicken-Liver, Eggplant and,
        124–125

Casserole(s) (continued)
    d'Agneau, 58–59
    Egg, Scalloped, Asparagus and,
        119
    Fountain-of-Youth, 134
    Harvest, 112–113
    Lamb and
        Macaroni, 60
        Spinach, 61
    Riz-Fromage, 144
    of Spinach, 128–129
Casserole d'Agneau, 58–59
Casserole Poulet aux Légumes, 72–
        73
Casserole of Spinach, 128–129
Céleri-Rave Hors d'Oeuvre, 24–25
Celery Cybele, 123
Celery Jelly, Asparagus in, 161
Cerises au Vin, 183
Cheese
    American Soufflé, 154–155
    and Eggs
        Andalusia, 149
        Baked Omelet, 149
        Daffodil, 150–151
        Frothy Asparagus, 152–153
        Nesting, 151–152
        Primavera, 150
        South-of-the-Border, 153
        Sunny Tomato, 154
    Lunar Custard, 157
    Pots of Gold, 156
    Spaghetti and Cheese Custard,
        157
    Strata, 156
    Sunday-Night Soufflé, 155
Cheese Appetizer (Alpine), 27
Cheese Canapés (Gold Fingers),
        214
Cheese Custard Hollande, 191
Cheese Custard, Spaghetti and, 157
Cheese and Pineapple Ring, 163
Cherry Float, 205
Chicken, 67–89
    -Avocado Appetizer, 26
    Baked, Sidney's, 76
    Beaumont Bake, 74

Chicken (*continued*)
  Breasts, Eden, 75
  Broiled, Sweet and Low, 70
  Capri, 73
  Casserole
    Chicken Noodle, 81
    Normandy, 80–81
    Poulet aux Légumes, 72–73
  -and-Cheese Strata, 83–84
  -Citron Mousse, 26–27
  Creamed, Mormi's, 79
  Custard, 25
  Dreams, 76–77
  and Eggs, Scalloped, 80
  Épinard, 83
  au Jus des Pommes, 74–75
  Liver(s)
    en Brochette, 84
    and Rice Casserole, 86–87
    Russian, 84–85
    Sherried, 86
    Supreme, 85
  with Peaches, 69
  Pilau of, 71
  Poulet en Aspic Rose, 78–79
  Roast Rumanian, 69
  Roulade, 82
  Sidney's Baked, 76
  Stew, Bruyère, 72
  -Stuffed Veal Roast, 63
  Tai-Pan, 77–78
  See also Poultry
Chicken-Avocado Appetizer, 26
Chicken Breasts Eden, 75
Chicken Capri, 73
Chicken-and-Cheese Strata, 83–84
Chicken-Citron Mousse, 26–27
Chicken Custard, 25
Chicken Dip, 214
Chicken Dreams, 76–77
Chicken Épinard, 83
Chicken au Jus des Pommes, 74–75
Chicken-Liver Casserole, Eggplant
    and, 124–125
Chicken Liver and Rice Casse-
    role, 86–87
Chicken Livers en Brochette, 84

Chicken Livers, Russian, 84–85
Chicken Livers, Sherried, 86
Chicken Livers Supreme, 85
Chicken Noodle Casserole, 81
Chicken with Peaches, 69
Chicken Roulade, 82
Chicken Salad Oahu, 163
Chicken Stew Bruyère, 72
Chicken-Stuffed Veal Roast, 63
Chicken Tai-Pan, 77–78
Chuck Roast, Hawaiian, 47
Classic Fruit Gelatin, 187
Cocktail Feuille Artichaut, 212
Cocktail Spread, Acapulco, 213
Coffee-Flavor Float, 206
Cold Pea Soup (Green Frappé), 38
Consommé mit Ei, 34–35
Cornish Hen in a Package, 87
Cranberry Ragout of Lamb, 59
Cream of Spinach Soup, 38–39
Cream of String Bean Soup, 39
Creamed Chicken, Mormi's, 79
Creamed Fillets, 96
Crème Brulée Facile, 188–189
Crunchy Apples, 181
Cucumber Soup, 35
Cucumbers, Scalloped, 124
Cucumbers, Stewed, 123
Custard, Cheese Hollande, 191
Custard, Chicken, 25
Custard, Lunar, 157
Custard with Meringues, 190
Custard, Moroccan, 191
Custard, Spaghetti and Cheese, 157

Daffodil Eggs, 150–151
Danish New Potatoes, 105
Danish Rice, 178
Dessert(s), 173–193
  Apricot Meringues, 175
  Apricot and Rice Pudding, 177–
    178
  Baked Pears, 185
  Banana Caribbean, 182
  Banana Honey, 182
  Basic Angel Food Cake, 174

Dessert(s) (continued)
    Caramel Riz Gâteau, 179
    Cerises au Vin, 183
    Cheese Custard Hollande, 191
    Classic Fruit Gelatin, 187
    Crème Brulée Facile, 188–189
    Crunchy Apples, 181
    Custard with Meringues, 190
    Danish Rice, 178
    Fruits Helène, 186
    Heavenly Banana Pudding, 192
    Homemade Banana Ice Cream,
        187–188
    Honolulu Peaches, 184
    Lemon Rice Puffs, 180–181
    Maple Cream, 189
    Moroccan Custard, 191
    Mousse El Exigente, 176–177
    Normandy Pudding, 192–193
    Orange Igloos, 184
    Pineapple Loaf, 185
    Plum Dandy, 186
    Prune-Whip Soufflé, 175
    Roman Parfait, 188
    Senator's Rice Pudding, 180
    Southern Banana Bake, 183
    Steamed Peach Soufflé, 176
    Tapioca el Hombre, 193
Dessert Sauce, New Orleans, 201
Deviled Eggs, Different, 215
Devonshire Illusion Sauce, 200
Diamond Head Potato Salad, 170
Different Deviled Eggs, 215
Dreamy Banana Malt, 204
Drinks and Shakes, 203–209
    Canario, 207
    Cherry Float, 205
    Coffee-Flavor Float, 206
    Dreamy Banana Malt, 204
    Holiday Eggnog, 208–209
    Long-Face Lifter, The, 209
    Maple Milk Shake, 207
    Oklahoma Shake, 205
    Pineapple Blossom, 207
    Secret Ingredient Banana
        Frosty, 204

Drinks and Shakes (continued)
    Strawberry Milk Shake, 208
    Superfruit Frosty, 208
    Tall, Tan, and Terriffic, 206
Duck, Rôti, lean, 88
Dutch Potatoes, 104

Easy Lemon Sauce, 201
Egg Aspic, Picnic, 165
Egg Casserole, Scalloped Aspara-
    gus and, 119
Egg Salad, Sicilian, 166
Egg and Tongue Salad, Jellied, 165
Eggnog, Holiday, 208–209
Eggplant and Chicken-Liver Cas-
    serole, 124–125
Eggplant, Scalloped, de Luxe, 125
Eggs Andalusia, 149
Eggs and Cheese, 147–157
    American Soufflé, 154–155
    Baked Omelet, 149
    Eggs
        Andalusia, 149
        Daffodil, 150–151
        Frothy Asparagus, 152–153
        Nesting, 151–152
        Primavera, 150
        South-of-the-Border, 153
        Sunny Tomato, 154
    Lunar Custard, 157
    Pots of Gold, 156
    Spaghetti and Cheese Custard,
        157
    Strata, 156
    Sunday-Night Soufflé, 155
Eggs, Daffodil, 150–151
Eggs, Deviled, Different, 215
Eggs, Frothy Asparagus, 152–153
Eggs Primavera, 150
Eggs, South-of-the-Border, 153
Eggs, Sunny Tomato, 154
Endives, Braised, 126–127
Endives Parisienne, 126
European Sauce Thickening
    Method, 197

Filets of Sole Vin Blanc Sec, 93
Fillets, Creamed, 96
First-Course Stuffed Tomatoes, 28–29
Fish, 91–101
  Boneless Red Snapper, 96
  Filets of Sole Vin Blanc Sec, 93–94
  Fillets, Creamed, 96
  Halibut
    Baked, au Gratin, 92
    Snowy Steaks, 92
  Paper-Baked Pompano, 93
  Puff, 100
  Rolls, Stuffed, 95
  Salmon
    Instant Hot, 98
    with Lemon Butter, Poached, 97
    and Rice Loaf, 98–99
    Soufflé, 99
    Steaks, Poached, 97
  Sole with Soufflé Sauce, 94
  Tuna Italiano, 100–101
  Turbans, 94–95
Fish Puff, 100
Fish Rolls, Stuffed, 95
Fish Salad, Stockholm, 166–167
Fish Turbans, 94–95
Float, Cherry, 205
Float, Coffee-Flavor, 206
Foie Gras Illusion, 215
Fountain-of-Youth Casserole, 134
Frothy Asparagus Eggs, 152–153
Fruit Gelatin, Classic, 187
Fruit-Juice Soup (Summer Luncheon), 36
Fruit Mold, Lamb and, 62
Fruits Helène, 186

Gazpacho Aspic, 28
Glazed Meat Loaf, 52–53
Gold Fingers, 214
Golden Mashed Potatoes, 109
Greek Soup, 34
Green Frappé, 38

Ground Beef, The Most Agreeable, 54–55
Ground Meat
  Glazed Meat Loaf, 52–53
  Hungarian Loaf, 64
  Meatballs Jutlandia, 52
  Most Agreeable Ground Beef, The, 54–55
  Polynesian Medley, 56–57
  Poorer-than-a-Shepherd Pie, 50–51
  Scandinavian Meat Ring, 51
  Tipsy Hamburgers, 54
  Toni's Meat Loaf, 54
  Veal-Tuna Loaf with Chicken Noodle Sauce, 64–65
  See also Meat (s)

Halibut, Baked, au Gratin, 92
Halibut Steaks, Snowy, 92
Hamburgers, Tipsy, 54
Harvest Casserole, 112–113
Hawaiian Chuck Roast, 47
Hearts of Palm, Minorcan, 127
Heavenly Banana Pudding, 192
High Spinach Soufflé, 129
Holiday Eggnog, 208–209
Hollandaise, Blender, 198
Homemade Banana Ice Cream, 187–188
Honey-Baked Acorn Squash, 130
Honey Gigot, 57
Honolulu Peaches, 184
Hostess Potatoes, 104
Hungarian Loaf, 64

Ice Cream, Banana, 192
Instant Hot Salmon, 98

Jellied Egg and Tongue, 165
Jellied Mandarin Orange and Lime Salad, 168

Lamb en Brochette, 58
Lamb, Cranberry Ragout of, 59
Lamb and Fruit Mold, 62

Lamb Kidneys Aloha, 65
Lamb and Marcaroni Casserole, 60
Lamb and Potatoes au Gratin,
    60–61
Lamb and Spinach Casserole, 61
Lean Duck Rôti, 88
Leftovers (Salad), 171
Lemon Rice Puffs, 180–181
Lemon Sauce, Easy, 201
Lime Salad, Jellied Mandarin
    Orange and, 168
Liver, see Calf's Liver; Chicken
    Livers
Long-Face Lifter, The, 209
Lunar Custard, 157

Macaroni Casserole, Lamb and, 60
Macaroni Luncheon Salad, 167
Macaroni Rarebit, 138
Macaroni-Salmon Salad, 168
Macaroni, Venetian, 137–138
Mandarin Orange and Lime
    Salad, Jellied, 168
Maple Cream, 189
Maple Milk Shake, 207
Mashed Potatoes, Golden, 109
Mayonnaise, Our Mandalay House,
    197
Meat(s), 41–66
    Beef
        Bohemian, 45
        Flamingo, 56
        Hawaiian Chuck Roast, 47
        Minsk, 49
        -Noodle Casserole, 55
        Viennese Boiled, 48
    Boeuf Bourguignon, Our Basic,
        48–49
    Boeuf en Gelée, 46–47
    Boiled Tomato Tongue, 66
    Calf's Liver, Broiled, 66
    Casserole d'Agneau, 58–59
    Chicken-Stuffed Veal Roast, 63
    Ground, see Ground Meat
    Hawaiian Chuck Roast, 47
    Honey Gigot, 57

Meat(s) (continued)
    Lamb
        en Brochette, 58
        Cranberry Ragout of, 59
        and Fruit Mold, 62
        Honey Gigot, 57
        and Macaroni Casserole, 60
        and Potatoes au Gratin, 60
        and Spinach Casserole, 61
    Lamb Kidneys Aloha, 65
    Meat Loaf
        Glazed, 52–53
        Hungarian, 64
        Toni's, 53
    Meatballs Jutlandia, 52
    Most Agreeable Ground Beef,
        54–55
    Polynesian Medley, 56–57
    Poorer-than-a-Shepherd Pie 50–
        51
    Scandinavian Meat Ring, 51
    Shepherd's Pie, 50
    Steak
        with Beef Marrow Sauce,
            44–45
        Parmigiana, 43
        Royal Bourbon, 44
        Sandwiches, 46
    Tipsy Hamburgers, 54
    Tongue, Boiled Tomato, 66
    Veal
        Hungarian Loaf, 64
        Veal Roast, Chicken Stuffed,
            63
        Veal-Tuna Loaf with Chicken
            Noodle Sauce, 64–65
Meatballs Jutlandia, 52
Meat Ring, Scandinavian, 51
Meringues, Apricot, 175
Meringues, with Custard, 190
Minorcan Hearts of Palm, 127
Minsk Beef, 49
Mormi's Creamed Chicken, 79
Moroccan Custard, 191
Most Agreeable Ground Beef, 54–
    55

Mousse, Avocado, 23
Mousse, Chicken-Citron, 26–27
Mousse El Exigente, 176–177

Nesting Eggs, 151–152
New Orleans Dessert Sauce, 201
New Potatoes and Beans, French Style, 106
New Potatoes, Danish, 105
Noodle Ring, Spring, 137
Normandy Chicken Casserole, 80
Normandy Pudding, 192–193
Norwegian Potato Pudding, 108

Oklahoma Shake, 205
Omelet, Baked, 149
Open Apple Rarebit, 22
Orange-Buttered Beets, 120
Orange Igloos, 184
Our Mandalay House Mayonnaise, 197

Paper-Baked Pompano, 93
Parfait, Roman, 188
Pasta, 135–145
  Baked Ravioli, 140–141
  Macaroni
    Rarebit, 138
    Venetian, 137–138
  Noodle Ring, Spring, 137
  Spaghetti
    au Gratin, 139
    la Scala, 139
    Soufflé, 140
  Spring Noodle Ring, 137
  See also Rice
Pea Purée, 128
Pea Soup (Green Frappé), 38
Peach, Steamed Soufflé, 176
Peaches, Honolulu, 184
Peaches, Pompeii, 169
Pears, Baked, 185
Picnic Egg Aspic, 165
Pilau of Chicken, 71
Pilgrim Squash, 130
Pineapple Blossom, 207
Pineapple Loaf, 185

Pineapple Ring, 169
Pineapple Ring, Cheese and, 163
Plum Dandy, 186
Poached Salmon, Lemon Butter, 97
Poached Salmon Steaks, 97
Polynesian Medley, 56–57
Poorer-than-a-Shepherd Pie, 50
Potato(es), 103–113
  Charlotte, 107
  Cheese Soufflé, 108
  Dutch, 104
  Harvest Casserole, 112–113
  Hostess, 104
  Killarney, 106–107
  Mashed Golden, 109
  New Potatoes
    and Beans, French Style, 106
    Danish, 105
  Scalloped, Milky Way, 105
  Sweet Potatoes
    Apple-Yam Dandy, 111
    de Luxe, 110
    Pudding, 110–111
    Sherried, 112
Potato Charlotte, 107
Potato Cheese Soufflé, 108
Potato Pudding, Norwegian, 108
Potato Salad, Diamond Head, 170
Potato Soup à la Maison, 36–37
Potatoes Killarney, 106–107
Pots of Gold, 156
Poulet en Aspic Rose, 78–79
Poultry, 67–89
  Cornish Hen in a Package, 87
  Lean Duck Rôti, 88
  Turkey in Champagne, 88–89
  Turkey Divan, 89
  see also Chicken
Prune-Whip Soufflé, 175
Pudding(s)
  Heavenly Banana, 192
  Normandy, 192–193
  Norwegian Potato, 108–109
  Sweet Potato, 110–111

Quick Spinach Sauce, 199

Rarebit, Macaroni, 138
Rarebit, Open Apple, 22
Ravioli, Baked, 140–141
Red Snapper, Boneless, 96
Rice, 141–145
  Arroz Redondo, 142
  Cajun, 145
  au Gratin in a Minute, 144
  Riz Rose, 142–143
  Riz-Fromage Casserole, 144
  and Tuna Pie, 143
  Yorkshire, 141
  See also Pasta
Rice au Gratin in a Minute, 144
Rice Loaf, Salmon and, 98–99
Rice Pudding, Apricot and, 177
Rice Pudding, Danish, 178
Rice Pudding, The Senator's, 180
Rice Puffs, Lemon, 180–181
Rice Salad (Salade Imperatrice), 164
Rice and Tuna Pie, 143
Riz Rose, 142–143
Riz-Fromage Casserole, 144
Roman Parfait, 188
Royal Bourbon Steak, 44
Rumanian Roast Chicken, 69
Russian Chicken Livers, 84–85
Russian Mold, 162

St. Patrick's Soup, 37
Salad(s), 159–171
  Asparagus in Celery Jelly, 161
  Asparagus Jockey Club, 162
  Black-and-White Molds, 170
  Cheese and Pineapple Ring, 163
  Chicken Salad Oahu, 163
  Diamond Head Potato Salad, 170
  Jellied Egg and Tongue, 165
  Jellied Mandarin Orange and Lime Salad, 168
  Macaroni Luncheon, 167
  Macaroni-Salmon, 168
  Peaches Pompeii, 169
  Picnic Egg Aspic, 165
  Pineapple Ring, 169

Salad(s) (*continued*)
  Russian Mold, 162
  Salade Imperatrice, 164
  Sicilian Egg, 166
  Stockholm Fish, 166–167
  Turkey-Cranberry Mold, 164
  Use-up-the-Leftovers, 171
Salade Imperatrice, 164
Salmon, Instant Hot, 98
Salmon with Lemon Butter, Poached, 97
Salmon-Macaroni Salad, 168
Salmon and Rice Loaf, 98–99
Salmon Soufflé, 99
Salmon Steaks, Poached, 97
Sardine Paté Canapés, 216
Sauce(s), 195–202
  Blender Hollandaise, 198
  Chicken Noodle, for Veal-Tuna Loaf, 64–65
  Devonshire Illusion, 200
  Easy Lemon, 201
  European Thickening Method, 197
  Mandalay House Mayonnaise, 197
  New Orleans Dessert, 201
  Quick Spinach, 199
  Sour Cream, 199
  Strawberry, 202
  Taste of Honey, 200
  Vanilla-Rum, 201
  Verte, 198
Scalloped Asparagus and Egg Casserole, 119
Scalloped Chicken and Eggs, 80
Scalloped Cucumbers, 124
Scalloped Eggplant de Luxe, 125
Scalloped Potatoes Milky Way, 105
Scandinavian Meat Ring, 51
Secret Ingredient Banana Frosty, 204
Senator's Rice Pudding, The, 180
Shakes and Drinks, 203–209
  Canario, 207
  Cherry Float, 205
  Coffee-Flavor Float, 206
  Dreamy Banana Malt, 204

Shakes and Drinks (continued)
  Holiday Eggnog, 208–209
  Long-Face Lifter, The, 209
  Maple Milk Shake, 207
  Oklahoma Shake, 205
  Pineapple Blossom, 207
  Secret Ingredient Banana, 204
  Strawberry Milk Shake, 208
  Superfruit Frosty, 208
  Tall, Tan, and Terrific, 206
Shepherd Pie, Poorer-than-a- 50–51
Shepherd's Pie, 50
Sherried Chicken Livers, 86
Sherried Sweet Potatoes, 112
Sicilian Egg Salad, 166
Sidney's Baked Chicken, 76
Snowy Halibut Steaks, 92
Sole with Soufflé Sauce, 94
Soufflé(s)
  American, 154–155
  High Spinach, 129
  Potato Cheese, 108
  Prune-Whip, 175
  Salmon, 99
  Spaghetti, 140
  Steamed Peach, 176
  Sunday-Night, 155
Soup(s), 21–40
  Alhambra, 40
  Avocado, 33
  Borscht in a Minute, 33
  Consommé mit Ei, 34–35
  Cream of Spinach, 38–39
  Cream of String Bean, 39
  Cucumber, 35
  à la Grecque, 34
  Green Frappé, 38
  Potato à la Maison, 36–37
  St. Patrick's, 37
  Summer Luncheon, 36
  Tomato Polevka, 40
Soup Alhambra, 40
Soup à la Grecque, 34
Sour Cream Sauce, 199
South-of-the-Border Eggs, 153
Southern Banana Bake, 183

Spaghetti and Cheese Custard, 157
Spaghetti au Gratin, 139
Spaghetti la Scala, 139
Spaghetti Soufflé, 140
Spinach Casserole, 128–129
Spinach Soufflé, High, 129
Spinach and Lamb Casserole, 61
Spinach and Potato Soup, 37
Spinach Primavera, 150
Spinach Sauce, Quick, 199
Spinach Soup, Cream of, 38–39
Spring Noodle Ring, 137
Squash, Acorn, Honey-Baked, 130
Squash Medley, 131
Squash, Pilgrim, 130
Squash with Asparagus, 118–119
Steak with Beef Marrow Sauce, 44–45
Steak Parmigiana, 43
Steak, Royal Bourbon, 44
Steak Sandwiches, 46
Steamed Peach Soufflé, 176
Stewed Cucumbers, 123
Stockholm Fish Salad, 166–167
Strata, 156
  Chicken-and-Cheese, 83–84
Strawberry Milk Shake, 208
Strawberry Sauce, 202
String Bean Soup, Cream of, 39
String Beans Mimosa, 132–133
Stuffed Fish Rolls, 95
Stuffed Tomatoes, First-Course, 28
Summer Luncheon Soup, 36
Sunday-Night Soufflé, 155
Sunny Tomato Eggs, 154
Superfruit Frosty, 208
Sweet and Low Broiled Chicken, 70
Sweet Potato(es)
  Apple-Yam Dandy, 111
  de Luxe, 110
  Harvest Casserole, 112–113
  Sherried, 112
Sweet Potato de Luxe, 110
Sweet Potato Pudding, 110–111

Tall, Tan, and Terrific, 206

226 - Index

Tapioca el Hombre, 193
Taste of Honey Dressing, 200
Tipsy Hamburgers, 54
Tomato Aspic (Gazpacho), 28
Tomatoes Stuffed, First Course, 28–29
Tomato Polevka, 40
Tomato Soup (Alhambra), 40
Tomato Stuffed with Broccoli, 133
Tomato, Sunny Eggs, 154
Tongue, Boiled Tomato, 66
Tongue, Jellied Egg and, 165
Toni's Meat Loaf, 53
Tuna-Avocado Cocktail Spread (Acapulco), 213
Tuna Italiano, 100–101
Tuna Pie, with Rice, 143
Tuna-Veal Loaf, with Chicken Noodle Sauce, 64–65
Turkey in Champagne, 88–89
Turkey-Cranberry Mold, 164
Turkey Divan, 89

Use-up-the-Leftovers Salad, 171

Vanilla-Rum Sauce, 201
Veal Roast, Chicken-Stuffed, 63
Veal-Tuna Loaf with Chicken Noodle Sauce, 64–65
Vegetable(s), 115–134
    Acorn Squash, 130
    Artichokes
        directions for cooking, 117
        à la Moscow, 22
        Saint Germain, 117–118
        à la Sidney, 118
    Asparagus
        Scalloped, Egg Casserole, 119
        with Summer Squash, 118
    Beets
        à la Crème, 120
        Orange-Buttered, 120
    Broccoli, Tomato Stuffed with, 133
    Carrots
        Glazed with Honey and Orange, 121

Vegetable(s) (continued)
    Hong Kong, 122
    The Very Best in the Whole World, 121
    Vichy, 122
    Celery Cybele, 123
    Cucumbers
        Scalloped, 124
        Stewed, 123
    Eggplant
        and Chicken-Liver Casserole, 124–125
        de Luxe, Scalloped, 125
    Endives
        Braised, 126–127
        Parisienne, 126
    Fountain-of-Youth Casserole, 134
    Hearts of Palm, Minorcan, 127
    Pea Purée, 128
    Spinach
        Casserole of, 128–129
        High Soufflé, 129
        Primavera, 150
    Squash
        Honey-Baked Acorn, 130
    Medley, 131
        Pilgrim, 130
        Summer, with Asparagus, 118
    String Beans Mimosa, 132–133
    Tomato Stuffed with Broccoli, 133
    Tomatoes, Stuffed, First Course, 28–29
    Zucchini
        Provençal, 131–132
        -Tomato Bake, 132
Venetian Macaroni, 137–138
Very Best Carrots in the Whole World, The, 121
Viennese Boiled Beef, 48

Yorkshire Rice, 141

Zucchini Provençal, 131–137
Zucchini-Tomato Bake, 132